ANTENATAL
AND POSTNATAL
DEPRESSION

XB   D0412460

ANTENATAL AND POSTNATAL DEPRESSION

Practical advice and support for all sufferers

Siobhan Curham

WOLVERHAMPTON PUBLIC LIBRARIES	
XB000000041410	
Bertrams	17/02/2010
618.76CUR	£9.99
P	709496

Vermilion
LONDON

3 5 7 9 10 8 6 4 2

Text © Siobhan Curham 2000
Illustrations © Ebury Press 2000

Siobhan Curham has asserted her right to be identified as the author of this
work under the Copyright, Designs and Patents Act 1988.

All rights reserved. No part of this publication may be reproduced,
stored in a retrieval system, or transmitted in any form or by any means,
electronic, mechanical, photocopying, recording or otherwise without the
prior permission of the copyright owners.

First published in 2000 by Vermilion, an imprint of Ebury Press
Random House, 20 Vauxhall Bridge Road, London SW1V 2SA

Random House Australia (Pty) Limited
20 Alfred Street, Milsons Point, Sydney
New South Wales 2061, Australia

Random House New Zealand Limited
18 Poland Road, Glenfield
Auckland 10, New Zealand

Random House (Pty) Limited
Isle of Houghton, Corner of Boundary Road & Carse O'Gowrie
Houghton 2198, South Africa

Random House Publishers India Private Limited
301 World Trade Tower, Hotel Intercontinental Grand Complex
Barakhamba Lane, New Delhi 110 001, India

The Random House Group Limited Reg. No. 954009

www.randomhouse.co.uk

A CIP catalogue for this book is available from the British Library

ISBN 9780091856076 (from January 2007)
ISBN 0091856078

Papers used by Vermilion are natural, recyclable products made from wood
grown in sustainable forests.

Printed and bound in Great Britain by Mackays of Chatham plc, Kent

Contents

Foreword

Everyone has heard of postnatal depression. About one in ten women is depressed in the first few weeks following childbirth. This is not the same as the severe but rare illness of postnatal psychosis, or the mild, common and transient condition called 'the blues'. Much less well known is that antenatal depression is just as common as postnatal depression. At any one time during pregnancy, about one in ten women will be depressed. About one in 30 will be depressed all through pregnancy and the postnatal period.

Actually about one in ten women of a similar age, who have *not* just had a baby, will be depressed too. Does this mean that antenatal and postnatal depression do not exist as specific conditions? Probably not. There do seem to be particular groups of women in whom becoming pregnant or giving birth does act as a specific trigger for depression. In others, the joy of the prospect of having a baby, or of giving birth, seems to protect them from the depression they would otherwise suffer. But depression is a very widespread problem.

We still know very little about the causes of either antenatal or postnatal depression. Most of us believe that the huge changes in levels of hormones such as oestrogen, chemicals that are known to have an effect on mood, must be something to do with it, but there is still very little hard evidence for this. There is evidence that psychological and social factors do play a role. Many studies have found that not having a supportive partner or other effective support network group, is definitely a risk factor, but it is not the whole story. Women with good relationships can be affected. A history of depression is also a risk factor. However, despite a lot of research our understanding is still quite limited. One reason for this is probably because there are many different causes, genetic, hormonal, psychological and social, and they operate to different degrees in different women.

Much recent research has focused on the effects on the child. And here there is increasing evidence that if the mother has post-natal depression the child, especially if it is a boy, can suffer from a lower IQ and behavioural problems. There is also some evidence to suggest that if the mother is anxious or depressed antenatally this can affect the development of the foetus, perhaps resulting in the child being less able to cope with stress later. These are not inevitable effects, and many children of mothers with depression will have no problems, but they highlight the importance of mothers with depression, either antenatal or postnatal, seeking help and treatment.

Here the picture is brighter. Depression is an eminently treatable disease. At the milder end it responds well to various types of 'talking' therapy. More severe depression can be effect-ively treated with antidepressants. We have recently carried out a small study which suggests that attending an infant massage class can help mothers with postnatal depression to relate better to their babies. What is very important is that mothers with either antenatal or postnatal depression should recognise the problem in themselves and then do something about it.

This is where this book has a real contribution to make. Siobhan Curham describes from the inside, by using many accounts taken from women who have experienced these condi-tions, what both antenatal and postnatal depression actually feel like. These, often moving, descriptions should make it easier for other women, and their partners, relatives or friends, to recognise and understand these common conditions. There is nothing to be ashamed of in suffering from depression, but women with these conditions probably cannot deal with it by themselves. They should seek help. This book will show them that they are not alone.

Vivette Glover DSc
Foetal and Neonatal Stress Research Centre,
Queen Charlotte's and Chelsea Hospital, London.
September 2000

Introduction

In this day and age of celebrity pregnancies, involving nude photo shoots and designer maternity wear, expecting a baby has never been so glamorous and exciting. At least that's what the world's media would have us believe. Yet beneath all of the see-through maternity smocks and Gucci baby slings the truth is that as many as 20 per cent of all mothers experience depression either before or immediately after the birth of their child.

When I discovered I was pregnant I was overjoyed, but by the time my baby was born I had turned into a nervous wreck. My relationship was at breaking point, I was unable to work and my confidence was at an all-time low. I was one of the 10 per cent of pregnant women who experience antenatal depression. I didn't realise this at the time – I didn't even know such a condition existed.

Although my pregnancy hadn't been planned my partner Colin and I were both really excited when we found out. We were very happy together, financially secure and ready to cope with the responsibilities of parenthood. At first the fact that I was pregnant brought us closer together. But then, just as my morning sickness began to subside and I started to look forward to the 'blooming' stage of pregnancy, I became the victim of uncontrollable crying fits. Any little thing would start me off – missing the bus, burning the toast – and I would be found in floods of tears. I had expected some kind of hormonal upheaval when I became pregnant and if this had been the extent of my mood swings I would have put up with it gladly, but unfortunately much worse was to come.

At some point in her pregnancy every woman worries about the health of her unborn child. In my case, however, these worries became inescapable, irrational fears. I would lie awake at night torturing myself with the memories of the alcohol I had consumed and the cigarettes I had smoked during the weeks before I realised I was pregnant. I read everything I could get my hands on about the damage this can cause to the foetus. Before long I had convinced myself that my baby would be born mentally or physically handicapped and it would be all my fault. I became terrified of giving birth and discovering the damage I had caused.

As I became consumed by fear my anxieties spilled over into other areas of my life. My career was the first to suffer. I worked in a sales environment and had previously thrived on the pressure of meeting targets. But my sleepless nights soon affected my performance and as my performance started to suffer so did my confidence. Every morning when the alarm went off I would be filled with dread; often I just couldn't face going in.

My work wasn't the only area in which I lost confidence. Before long my friendships started to suffer too. I became convinced that my friends would no longer want to know me now that I had forgotten how to have fun. Some days I would lie on my bed, curled up in a ball, refusing to answer the phone or open the door when people called. All I wanted to do was to be alone and cry.

The worst casualty of my depression was my relationship with my partner Colin. I became convinced that he was about to leave me. If he went out with his friends I was sure that he was out meeting other women – slimmer, happier women. I turned from an easy-going, fun-loving partner into a possessive, paranoid wreck. Despite all of his reassurances to the contrary I became convinced that our relationship was doomed before our baby had even arrived.

At this point I really felt I could no longer go on and started to doubt my ability as a mother. How could I take care of a new life when I was finding it so hard to cope with my own? I spent hours searching through pregnancy books and magazines in the hope of finding some kind of explanation or reassurance, but to no avail.

I felt completely alone and was too scared to ask for help for fear that my doctor or midwife would think me unfit to be a mother.

Then my son was born. Despite all my fears to the contrary he was completely healthy and his arrival immediately brought Colin and me closer together again. However, it took about three months for my depression to disappear completely, as I struggled with exhaustion, the joys of breast-feeding, and worrying myself sick about whether I was doing everything right. A celebrity-style photo shoot of mother and baby 'relaxing at home' would have made for some pretty scary viewing in those first few weeks! Eventually however, I returned to my old self, but I was still very confused by what had happened to me. I had no previous history of depression and every time I heard somebody talking about the joys of pregnancy I felt that I had somehow been cheated.

It is now three years since I gave birth and in that time I have learnt a great deal about antenatal and postnatal depression. Recent research has proved that antenatal depression can affect the foetus, in some cases causing low birth weight and even premature delivery. One-third of all cases of postnatal depression actually begin during pregnancy and yet there is no literature or support group available to sufferers.

This is the book that I was searching for when I was pregnant. I have tried to answer all of the questions that I asked and have since been asked. Using other women's experiences I have examined the different causes of antenatal and postnatal depression and looked at the links between the two. As there are some important similarities and connections between the two types of depression I would recommend that sufferers of either read both sections. This book offers advice that is both practical and safe and also highlights the preventative steps that can be taken. Above all, in writing this book I want to reassure sufferers of antenatal and postnatal depression that they are certainly not alone and should never feel too ashamed or afraid to seek help.

Chapter 1
Antenatal Depression

What is Antenatal Depression?

Until very recently the only form of depression associated with pregnancy was postnatal. But in the last ten years many studies have been carried out on antenatal depression and its effects upon the foetus. These studies have shown that 10 per cent of pregnant women are affected by antenatal depression. More worryingly, they have also proved that stress and anxiety in the mother may be transmitted to the unborn child. This in turn has been linked to low birth weight, premature birth and all the long term health implications these entail.

The causes of antenatal depression are many and often complex. Women who do seek help are often told not to worry – *'it's just your hormones'* – but this is far too simplistic and of little help to the sufferer. The causes can be broken down into three main areas and may often be a combination of the following:

- **Physical**
- **Emotional**
- **Social**

The reality of antenatal depression

Doom, despondency and despair are not words normally associated with pregnancy, yet for the sufferer of antenatal depression they are all too familiar. Rather than being a time for hope, joy or blooming, pregnancy becomes a nine-month tunnel of gloom, depression and often ill health. Rather than knitting booties, choosing names and decorating nurseries it becomes a time for fear, anxiety and even contemplating suicide, as the following examples demonstrate:

Hannah's story

'Despite planning our pregnancy, both my husband and myself have been shocked at how immediate the conception was, which resulted in instant feelings of despair and depression. The whole nine months were not totally negative but more often than not I found myself in floods of tears, feeling total despondency, fear and helplessness without knowing "WHY?" I had a normal, uncomplicated pregnancy, secure relationship, was financially comfortable, but did not enjoy at all the journey to motherhood.'

Jane's story

'When I was pregnant with my daughter Emily, now 3 years, 9 months, I worried about everything. I had only been going out with my partner for five months when I found out I was pregnant. After the initial excitement wore off I began to get anxious about everything. At seven weeks pregnant I started to bleed. I was sent to the hospital for an internal scan which revealed the blood was coming from outside the womb and not to worry, but all I could think about was that I might lose my baby and if I did my partner would not want to marry me or know me any more. My fears were totally unfounded as I didn't miscarry – even though I bled up until 25 weeks pregnant. As I got bigger I was consumed with the fear of being alone, so I ended up spending most of my time with my mum. I had also been plagued with water infections which made me even more depressed. In the end I ended up having Emily five weeks early as a water infection caused *premature labour. Luckily she was born a healthy 2.9kg (6lb 7oz) and with no breathing difficulties so we were allowed home after three days. But I went on to develop postnatal depression.'*

Sara's story

'I didn't find out I was pregnant until I was 20 weeks. I was on the pill and still having periods so I had no idea. I'm 21 years old and this is my first baby. I am in a stable relationship and my partner is very supportive, but I'm having a very hard time being positive about this pregnancy. I love my partner, it's just everyone else I can't cope with. I'm being offered advice and opinions from people who have never had children. I've lost all of my self-confidence and I feel so lonely. It's as if my life and body have been taken over and I have no control any more. I'm glad to know that soon there may be some more support for other people who feel this way, which may take away some of the loneliness.'

Nicola's story

'I had this kind of depression for ages; I couldn't stop crying over anything sad that I'd see on the television or any little thing at all. I looked and felt a mess – bloom in pregnancy – that's a joke! I felt like all of my friends and family had moved on and left me behind. It was like I had a split personality – fine one minute and like a mad woman the next – and I was terrified my baby would be born a nervous wreck. I was not like this with either of my other pregnancies and my partner, Tom, thought I was an absolute nutter, as I felt if I let him do anything on his own away from me he was going to meet someone else, and that would have absolutely destroyed me. All the reassurance in the world didn't help me. I didn't look into my feelings as I was scared I was somehow abnormal.'

Common symptoms of antenatal depression

- **Chronic anxiety**
  Such as fear of the birth itself or fear for the baby's health
- **Guilt**
  Guilt at negative feelings towards the pregnancy
  Torturing oneself over any alcohol and cigarettes consumed during the pregnancy
- **Incessant crying**
  Often for no apparent reason
- **Lethargy**
  Lack of energy or enthusiasm for anything, including work, socialising and relationships
- **Loss of self-confidence**
  Often linked to changing body shape
- **Relationship problems**
  Acute fear that your partner is going to leave you, extreme possessiveness
- **Conflict with parents**
  The prospect of becoming a parent can often highlight difficulties with your own parents, particularly your mother
- **Isolation**
  Believing that you are the only one experiencing such feelings
- **Afraid to seek help**
  Too embarrassed and ashamed, for fear that you will be judged unfit to be a mother

Antenatal Depression
– the Physical Causes

Imagine if, one day before you ever became pregnant, you woke up and found that you had gained over 12.6kg (2 stone) in weight and your breasts had swollen to the size of two painful melons. You leap out of bed in horror only to collapse to the floor overcome by dizziness and nausea. Your bladder feels as if it is about to burst and you rush to the bathroom. No sooner have you relieved yourself than you need to go again. You look in your wardrobe for something to wear, but nothing fits any more apart from that old pair of leggings and that tatty old jumper you wore to do the decorating. You walk downstairs and are left gasping for breath because your lungs (and all your other internal organs) have been pushed right up inside your ribcage. Your heart is working 40 per cent harder than normal and your hormone levels – well they have rocketed.

This might sound like a nightmare but this is the biological reality of pregnancy. It is not really surprising therefore that such a physical trauma can often lead to feelings of depression and despair.

Hormonal changes

During pregnancy the hormones oestrogen and progesterone rise in volume by 30–50 times. The immediate effects of this are an increased need to urinate, breast swelling and morning sickness. In a normal pregnancy these increases should also create a sense of well-being, or the traditional maternal 'bloom'. However, in some pregnancies the placenta does not produce enough of the hormone progesterone. Although this does not affect the baby it can lead to feelings of depression in the mother.

Angela, 35, did not discover she was expecting a baby until she was five months pregnant. Despite having had no morning sickness or any of the other physical symptoms associated with pregnancy she suddenly became depressed for no apparent reason.

'Before I found out I was pregnant I was terrible; I kept not turning up at work as I didn't want to face anyone. I didn't want to see people, answer the phone or door and kept crying over the silliest things.'

This was soon having a serious impact on Angela's marriage:

> 'I had also become completely obsessed with cleaning and everything had to be just so. I'd get really upset if anyone changed my routine. In fact on one occasion I even hit my husband for taking the Hoover away from me. It got so bad my husband said if I didn't sort myself out it would seriously affect our relationship.'

So Angela went along to the doctors thinking she was going through an early menopause. It was only when the doctor sent her for a scan, suspecting she might be suffering from an ovarian cyst, that they discovered she was pregnant. The fact that Angela had no idea she was expecting demonstrates the impact that hormonal changes can have on a woman's mental well-being.

Chronic nausea

One side effect of a hormone imbalance is chronic nausea. For a lot of women there is no such thing as 'morning' sickness. It lasts all day and often for the whole nine months. Permanently feeling sick can cause feelings of utter despair as Eleanor, 31, discovered when pregnant with her eldest daughter Kate.

> 'From practically the moment Kate was conceived right up until I gave birth I felt sick. People don't realise just how much this affects your day-to-day life. One morning I was sick on the train going to work – it was awful – everybody was staring at me. I became too scared to go in, and even when I did make it into the office I wasn't much use to anyone as I spent more time in the toilet than at my desk.'

Work was not the only area of Eleanor's life to be affected. Her sickness prevented her from going out with friends and she became increasingly frustrated and depressed.

'I felt as if I had been pregnant forever – I really couldn't imagine feeling normal again, enjoying food and being able to smell things like coffee without wanting to heave.'

Alison, a nursery nurse, loved her job and wanted to carry on working right up until the birth of her child. However, chronic sickness forced her to leave work very early on in her pregnancy.

'I loved working with children and having to give up was the trigger for me becoming seriously depressed. Without the social aspect of going out to work and mixing with other people I lost all my enthusiasm for life and indeed my pregnancy.'

As with premenstrual tension and period pains, morning sickness is one of those 'women's complaints' that receives little sympathy from society in general and men in particular. It is looked upon as part and parcel of being a woman and sufferers are expected just to carry on and endure it in silence. However, chronic nausea over a long period of time is extremely unpleasant and can make life quite unbearable. For further information on the treatment of chronic nausea please see the chapters on diet and alternative therapies later on in this book.

Iron and zinc deficiency

Deficiencies in the minerals iron and zinc have both been linked to depression. As pregnancy is a common cause of such deficiencies it is crucial that the diet is full of iron- and zinc-rich foods (see Chapter 7 for examples of such foods). Vitamin C is also essential as this aids the absorption of iron into the body. Routine antenatal blood tests will detect iron deficiency and high dosage iron tablets will be prescribed. Sinead describes her feeling of relief when chronic anaemia was diagnosed during her first pregnancy:

'There was no way that my first child was unwanted or unplanned. Ever since I was a young girl I had longed to be a mother, so discovering I was pregnant was like a dream come true. However, after about three months I felt dreadful. I'm usually a real get-up-and-go sort of person, but I was constantly tired, ratty and miserable. I looked and felt terrible. I hated feeling so low at a time when I knew I should have been really excited. One day, when I was shopping in my local supermarket, I bent down to take something off the bottom shelf and I practically blacked out. I had never felt so dizzy before in my life and I was literally seeing stars before my eyes. It was a very frightening experience. I went to see my GP and he immediately suggested that I might be suffering from anaemia. So I had a blood test and he was right – my iron levels were very low and I was put on iron supplements. My midwife was also very helpful and gave me a list of foods that are rich in iron. Although it took a while before I noticed any improvement it was a huge relief to have an explanation for the way I had been feeling, and one that was relatively easy to put right.'

Weight gain

None of us like gaining weight and yet in pregnancy we are expected to put on at least 12.6kg (2 stone) and feel radiant about it! Excessive weight gain can have a profound effect upon a woman's confidence, leading to feelings of worthlessness and low self-esteem. Natalie, 28, had always been a size 8 until she became pregnant and grew to a size 16. Previously the life and soul of any party, as her confidence diminished she became increasingly moody and tearful.

'Before I became pregnant I lived for the weekends when I would hit the clubs with my friends. I loved dancing and showing off my figure – I was one of the girls. But then I got

pregnant and it seemed as if my whole life came to an end. We had planned the pregnancy and I had been so excited at first. I thought I'd be able to carry on going out, obviously not drinking or smoking any more, but I still thought I'd be able to have a good old dance. However, within a couple of months I had just ballooned. I'd never had a problem with my weight before, but now I just couldn't seem to stop putting it on. It was all over as well – not just my stomach. I felt like a monster next to my slim mates. I stopped going out and this made me even more miserable. My husband became really distant and I was convinced this was because he no longer found me attractive, when the reality was that he was too scared to come near me in case he got his head bitten off.'

Suzanne's depression got worse and worse the larger she became:

'My "bump" continued to grow, and nothing in my wardrobe fitted, which added to my feelings of helplessness. Sometimes I would stay in my nightie all day because I just didn't see the point in getting dressed or doing anything. All the books said what a happy and exciting time this should be, but I felt fat and frumpy; a great big useless Easter egg on legs!'

As well as affecting confidence, excessive weight gain is also extremely uncomfortable. By the last two months of any pregnancy the simplest things, like walking up a flight of stairs, become major challenges. For previously active women this can prove extremely frustrating and lead to feelings of utter hopelessness, as Lucy recalls:

'I enjoyed most of my pregnancy but by the last couple of months everything changed. I became desperate. I hated what I had turned into. I felt like a gigantic blob, huffing and puffing along. Even getting out of a chair had become a struggle and I dreaded having to leave the house. I remember making

myself run up and down the stairs in the hope that I might go into labour early – all I could think about was getting this thing out of me. I know that's an awful way to talk about my own child, but I had become so resentful at having my body taken over.'

Physical complications during pregnancy

Pregnancy is a physical trauma in itself, but if there are added complications it is hardly surprising that the mother becomes consumed with anxiety, for her baby's health as well as her own. Sandra recounts how physical complications in her third pregnancy caused her to fear for her own sanity:

'I had been feeling quite down, for no apparent reason, throughout my pregnancy and then suddenly I went into labour at 25 weeks. I was admitted to hospital and given two doses of steroid injections over the space of 12 hours to mature the baby's lungs. Luckily it all stopped. The scans showed the baby was okay and weighed at the time about 1.2kg (2¹/₂lb). Then I was found to have a bad infection and was passing blood, so I was put on antibiotics. My symptoms led them to do a sugar level test for diabetes. The level should have been 6; mine was 12.5 so I had to go back into hospital for more tests. All this stress did little for my sanity and I spent the remainder of my pregnancy seriously believing I would end up on the psychiatric ward.'

Annabel suffered from antenatal depression during her first pregnancy and like Sandra it was exacerbated by the physical problems she encountered:

'All through my pregnancy, right from before I knew, I had these really bad pains about once a month. They were just below my right bottom rib and it was not until I was 32 weeks

that I was diagnosed as having gall stones. The pain was so bad that I was admitted into hospital. I was put on a women's surgical ward along with ladies who had had hysterectomies and a young girl who was having an early pregnancy bleed. This made me even more depressed, and if I had not been pregnant I would have killed myself as the pain was that bad. They gave me Pethidine but even this was not strong enough; they couldn't give me anything else because of the baby. All this worry was making life with my husband unbearable, he just didn't understand what I was going through. Everyone else I talked to just said I was being silly and to get on with it. This did not help me and just left me feeling even more alone.'

There are various complications that can be triggered off or made worse by pregnancy. If you start to feel any kind of pain or discomfort or notice any strange symptoms whilst you are pregnant it is imperative that you seek medical advice immediately. Although traditional treatments may not be available because of the unknown risk to the foetus, your doctor or midwife should be able to offer something to alleviate the symptoms and make life as comfortable as possible for you and your baby.

Antenatal Depression
– the Emotional Causes

All too often sufferers of antenatal depression are told that their mood swings are due to their hormones and there is very little that can be done to help. This, however, completely ignores the emotional impact of pregnancy. Whether it is for the first or the fifth time, planned or by accident, the responsibility of bringing a new life into the world should never be underestimated.

The first-time pregnancy involves a complete change of status; you are no longer just somebody's daughter, sister or aunt, you are about to become somebody's mother, and this prospect can be extremely daunting. It can also throw any number of skeletons out of the closet. Problems with your partner or even your own parents suddenly become magnified. Relationships with friends can change overnight, particularly if they are still young, free and childless. This in turn can lead to a loss of self confidence and feelings of inadequacy. Even if you are already a parent, a new pregnancy can cause a huge upheaval; the fear of how you will cope with another child, especially as you become more tired, can cause feelings of despair.

Virtually every sufferer of antenatal depression seems to be haunted by some form of chronic anxiety. This can be anything from concern for the baby's health to fear of the birth itself; from doubting your ability to be a good mother to extreme possessiveness over your partner. In many cases it is difficult to tell if these anxieties are a symptom or in fact the cause of antenatal depression, but either way they certainly need to be addressed.

The first-time pregnancy

Although Lisa and her husband Steve had decided to stop using birth control they had assumed it would take at least a year for Lisa to conceive. When she became pregnant virtually straight away Lisa was horrified.

> 'The minute I saw that blue line I thought to myself, "My God, what have I done?" I felt like a 16-year-old kid who had got herself into trouble rather than a happily married woman of 30.'

Lisa had never suffered from any form of depression before and yet suddenly she felt a complete sense of desolation:

> 'I was constantly calling myself stupid for getting pregnant. My self-esteem just hit rock bottom. Some days I couldn't

even get out of bed I felt so low. Little things like ironing or cleaning seemed impossible and that made me feel even more of a failure.'

When Lisa eventually told her GP how she was feeling he referred her to Queen Charlotte's Hospital in London for counselling. It was during one of Lisa's counselling sessions that she likened her pregnancy to how she had felt when her father died. In many cases first-time pregnancy can be very similar to a state of mourning – instead of blooming, mothers find themselves grieving for their loss of independence. This is particularly true for younger women.

Beth was just 16 years old when she became pregnant. Although previously she had always thought a baby would make her life complete, the reality was somewhat different:

'I felt that to be a responsible mother I would have to give up my entire social life. I completely disassociated myself from all of my friends, and my social life, which had previously consisted of going out drinking, smoking and clubbing, was reduced to me withdrawing totally.'

The most important thing to remember during a first-time pregnancy is that you are not going to be pregnant forever (although at times it can certainly feel like it). Once the baby is born you immediately get your body back to yourself, and it is not long before you start to get your life back too. Being able actually to see and hold your baby makes a huge difference. As you bond with your baby you will probably experience feelings you never knew existed – and that's not just new levels of exhaustion! Beth's baby is now nearly a year old and she is enjoying every moment of being a mum.

'I go to college part-time and I still see a lot of my friends, but the best thing is coming home to my son. I love being a mum to him.'

The unplanned pregnancy

Sharon, 21, was on the pill and still having periods when she discovered she was 20 weeks pregnant. Although she was in a loving, stable relationship the shock of being pregnant and the changes it meant to her life brought on extreme feelings of depression:

> 'I can't stand to be around anyone; anything people say to me seems to annoy or upset me. I feel like everyone thinks they know what's best for me. People treat me as if I'm stupid. I hate what's happening to my body; I've lost all my confidence and although I feel so lonely I hate everyone around me apart from my partner. I'm beginning to feel quite resentful, I'm scared I won't love our baby once it's born and I feel totally alone. I detest being pregnant – I hate everything about it. I just want my life back and my body back, but I know it can't happen.'

Becoming pregnant brings dramatic changes to a woman's life, even when it has been planned with military precision, but to become pregnant by accident has a huge impact. Your whole life has to be redefined and there is very little time in which to do so. It is essential that you make the most of the time before the baby arrives to come to terms with what has happened. Learn all you can about becoming a mother and seek support from those closest to you (particularly those with children).

Previous miscarriage or stillbirth

If you have suffered the tragedy of losing a child to miscarriage or stillbirth it is inevitable that any subsequent pregnancies will be fraught with the anxiety that it will happen again. It is not just this anxiety that can lead to antenatal depression; becoming pregnant again can also arouse deep feelings of loss as you find yourself mourning all over again for the child that died. Jane talks of the pain she went through following the loss of her second child:

> 'During my second pregnancy I didn't suffer from antenatal depression, but at 13½ weeks fate dealt me a dreadful blow when my scan showed that my baby had died. I was so depressed after this that I tried to kill myself by cutting my wrists and taking an overdose. I spent a week in a psychiatric ward and was diagnosed as having suffered a nervous breakdown. Last year I found myself pregnant again. I suffered antenatal depression throughout the whole pregnancy. I convinced myself that this baby would die and I would often cry myself to sleep thinking about it. If there was a sad item on the news I would cry bucketsful of tears. I was so highly strung that I refused to drive for the whole nine months for fear that something might happen, as I had no confidence in my own abilities during this time. After a quick, induced labour my baby was born a healthy 4.2kg (9lb 8oz). Although I still went on to develop postnatal depression it wasn't nearly as bad as I was given progesterone pessaries for the first 6–8 weeks which dramatically helped to reduce the depression. Even though I would like more children, I couldn't go through the anxiety of another pregnancy. Not only is it exhausting, it can cause a rift in your relationship with your husband or partner. Luckily I have a very patient and caring husband who has stood by me, even though at times I didn't want him around as I wanted to wallow in self-pity.'

It is hard to comprehend the pain and fear that women like Jane go through following the loss of a baby. Any subsequent pregnancy is bound to be a highly emotional experience; the joy of expecting another baby can easily be overshadowed by a sense of loss and a fear of history repeating itself. If you are in a similar situation to Jane discuss your fears with your midwife or GP, who may refer you to a trained counsellor for further advice and support.

Chronic anxieties

Virtually without exception every case of antenatal depression seems to manifest itself in some form of chronic anxiety. These anxieties can be very different, but they all leave the sufferer frantic with worry and extremely afraid, as the following examples will demonstrate.

'I'll never make a good mum'

Emma describes her pregnancy two years ago as 'mental torture; a roller-coaster of fear and depression'. Having become pregnant with twins at her first attempt at IVF treatment her initial happiness soon disappeared as she became obsessed with what kind of mother she would make.

> *'I was always calling up my friends to ask questions. What sort of nappies should I buy? What do I do if the baby falls asleep while breast feeding? When, precisely, do you put a baby in real clothes during the day? It was terrible, the pressure kept building up in my head. I never actually thought that I would do anything to my babies or to myself but I didn't know how I could carry on. I was desperate – I even thought of phoning the Samaritans.'*

Emma eventually confided in her yoga instructor who put her in touch with a counsellor midwife. Although counselling did not completely cure Emma of her depression it put her back on the right track:

> *'Ann told me the one thing I wanted to hear. She said the depression would pass. I was not mad. I think she gave me the first glimmer of joy.'*

Another important point to remember here is that for thousands upon thousands of years women have managed quite adequately to bring children into the world without the help of instruction books and leaflets, videos and workshops, and in many places they are still doing so today. Perhaps the fact that we are so bombarded with information has caused us to be almost blinded by science, and in some cases panic, forgetting just how natural a process reproduction is. As with all natural things parenthood is part trial and error, part instinct and part closing your eyes and just hoping for the best.

'My partner is going to leave me'

Perhaps because of the physical changes involved in pregnancy, a large proportion of sufferers of antenatal depression become convinced that their partners are going to leave them.

When Nicola was pregnant with her first child by her new partner she became terrified that he would meet somebody else.

> *'John's a couple of years younger than me and although that had never been an issue before, the minute I became pregnant it was all I could think about. I would spend hours at home picturing him meeting other women at the shop where he works. I would find any excuse to come and visit him, trying to catch him out. For the first time in my life I needed constant reassurance that he loved me, but John isn't like that – he's a real man's man and he finds it really hard to show his feelings.'*

Charlene, 21, spent the whole of her first pregnancy wrestling with similar feelings of possessiveness:

> *'For the first time ever I'm so paranoid and insecure about my partner. I know he loves me and I know he's totally faithful, however I can't help these ridiculous feelings. I'm scared that once the baby's born I'll be jealous of the time it takes up with my partner.'*

One aspect of pregnancy that often goes unmentioned is the effect it has on the father. Your partner is probably going through all the same feelings of nervousness, apprehension and excitement as the big day looms. However low you may be feeling about yourself you are the mother of his unborn child and this should never be underestimated. Of course there are some men who are unfaithful to their partners while they are pregnant, but these are the men who would probably be unfaithful anyway. In the vast majority of cases of this type of antenatal anxiety the woman's fears are completely unfounded and due purely to a lack of self-esteem. Rather than wasting valuable time interrogating him about why he's late home from work, or rifling through his pockets for that tell-tale receipt, you should concentrate on rebuilding your own self confidence.

'I'm terrified of the birth'

Linda suffered from antenatal depression during both her pregnancies and both times she became convinced she would die in childbirth.

> 'During my first pregnancy I felt absolutely certain that something terrible was going to happen during the birth. If I didn't die I was sure that the baby would. This fear was made even worse when I saw one of those real birth videos called "Stephanie's Labour" at the hospital. I was mortified and I demanded to be booked in for a caesarean; when this was refused I demanded counselling.'

Although her first labour went smoothly, Linda found herself experiencing all the same fears during her second pregnancy:

> 'When I was pregnant with my daughter I suffered from the most horrific recurrent nightmares. They were like something from the film "Rosemary's Baby". I started to believe that my baby was evil; that it was going to kill me.'

Fear of labour is understandable, particularly during the first pregnancy when you have no idea what to expect. It is important to remember that in this day and age of advanced techniques and well-trained staff there is no reason to let a natural sense of apprehension turn into feelings of terror. If fear of the birth is beginning to take over your life seek help and reassurance from your doctor or midwife. There are a wide range of treatments and techniques available to help provide a stress-free labour, such as hypnotherapy, acupuncture, aromatherapy and yoga.

'I know there's something wrong with my baby'

It is only natural for an expectant mother to worry about the health of her unborn child. In a normal pregnancy these fears are usually fleeting, with satisfactory scan results bringing reassurance. However, if you are suffering from antenatal depression all the scans in the world will never remove the nagging fear that something is wrong, as Angela discovered:

> *'Things were made worse by the fact that my 12-week scan was approaching fast. What if there is something wrong with the baby? This was the only thing that I could think about. I was constantly ratty, miserable and depressed and just didn't know what to do. When I had my scan they told me everything was fine and the baby was growing well, but even this did not stop me worrying. Even when I had my 20-week scan and they had done all the measurements I still worried that there was something they might have missed. As my pregnancy progressed everyone kept telling me, "You must be so happy, it won't be long now until the baby is here." But my fears were still growing: maybe the drugs they had given me had harmed the baby; maybe I have eaten something I shouldn't have; what if it has a hare lip? I knew I wouldn't be sure until it was all over and the baby was born.'*

A large proportion of pregnancies are unplanned and inevitably there are will be a few weeks (and in some cases months) when the mother may be drinking or smoking before realising she is pregnant. These weeks often come back to haunt sufferers of antenatal depression, who will read anything they can get their hands on about the damage they may have caused the foetus. Although drinking and smoking in pregnancy are certainly not advisable it is important to keep things in perspective. As long as you are careful from the moment you learn you are pregnant there is no reason why you should not go on to give birth to a perfectly healthy child, as Angela discovered:

'The day I had Alana was the greatest day of my life. She was perfect in every way; all my fears about something being wrong disappeared. All I had to worry about now was getting through the sleepless nights and her growing up and all the problems that brings!'

'How will I cope with twins?'

All expectant mothers of multiple births must wonder how on earth they will cope with the demands of more than one new baby, but for sufferers of antenatal depression the prospect of twins can seem quite unbearable, as Mrs Stevenson quickly discovered:

'I suffered from antenatal depression all through my pregnancy, from six weeks right up until the birth. The strange thing was that my husband and I had been trying for a baby for six years and I eventually fell pregnant through IVF treatment. I think part of my problem was that I conceived twins and was just so frightened of how I would cope. I'm a fairly open person, but found that people didn't understand – they thought I should be pleased I was finally pregnant. So I didn't say any more to anybody. I couldn't make sense of it, and at times I even found myself hoping that I would only manage to carry one baby.'

Although twins are obviously harder work than just one baby there is a danger in over-emphasising just how much harder. New babies all cause sleepless nights and feelings of exhaustion, whether you are contending with one or three. However, once the first few weeks are over the benefits of having twins will start to come to the fore, as Mrs Stevenson realised:

> *'The twins are three months old now and I can honestly say these last three months have been brilliant. I had geared myself up for such a hard time when they came, but it was nowhere near as bad as I had expected. They truly are good babies.'*

'I feel like I'm going mad'

> *'I feel like I'm going mad'; 'I started to believe I was destined for the psychiatric ward'; 'What the hell is wrong with me?'; 'I thought I was the only person in the world to have gone through this.'*

These are just some examples of the real fear for their own sanity that sufferers of antenatal depression have expressed to me. The lack of publicity and support available can make antenatal depression a terrifying experience. Unaware that 10 per cent of other pregnant women are going through exactly the same thing, sufferers fear that they are cracking up. It becomes impossible to imagine that one day they will return to their normal selves. Women are left feeling isolated and ashamed, with fear for their own mental health adding to all their other anxieties. The good news is that as more research is carried out into the effects of antenatal depression, public, and indeed medical, awareness will hopefully be raised in an attempt to conquer this illness.

Antenatal Depression
– the Social Causes

When I told my friend's grandmother that I was writing a book on antenatal and postnatal depression she sniffed loudly and informed me rather haughtily that, 'We didn't have things like that in our day

– we just got on with it'. Antenatal depression was only just beginning to be recognised in the 1990s, but it is unclear whether it is actually a relatively new phenomenon. We are certainly encouraged to express our feelings more these days, so perhaps previous generations of expectant mothers simply felt unable to admit what they were going through. However, other important social changes have undoubtedly placed pregnant women under increasing pressure, leaving them far more prone to depression.

The breakdown of the extended family

Gone are the days of three, sometimes four generations of the same family living side by side. Nowadays families are shrinking rapidly and living further and further apart. This is not always such a bad thing, as countless mother-in-law jokes will testify. However, when it comes to pregnancy there is a lot to be said for having a support network of female relatives on hand offering help and advice.

Shelly puts her antenatal depression down to the fact that her parents had returned to their native Australia by the time she first became pregnant:

'I was born and raised in England, but when I was 24 my parents returned to Australia. Although I obviously missed them their going didn't really affect my life too badly, I was happily married and had a terrific job. Yet when I became pregnant it all changed. I missed my mum so much and I dreaded giving birth. I really couldn't see how I would cope without her there to help me, to show me how to do the basic things like changing a nappy or breast-feed correctly. It felt like I spent the whole of my pregnancy crying for my parents; I felt just like a little child again.'

The changing role of women at work

A well-known popstar recently declared that the impending birth of her child would not affect her career, nor would she employ a nanny to assist her in her maternal role. She would be a fully hands-on mother whilst working full-time in the recording studio or on the road. Although this show of confidence and optimism was indeed admirable (if not a little naïve) pregnancy can send many a successful career woman into a state of panic. Women are under greater pressure than ever before to succeed in the world of work, so the additional pressures that pregnancy brings can often lead to feelings of despair. Maria was working as an account manager when she became pregnant with her first child:

'My pregnancy was totally unplanned, but I was quite excited when I first discovered I was expecting. However, as time went by I started to get more and more resentful. I had spent years getting to my position at work and I have to admit I got a real buzz from the money and the lifestyle that went with it. I felt proud to be a success in a male-dominated area, but my pregnancy threw me into a state of confusion. I felt torn between wanting to achieve more success in my career and my growing maternal instincts. I knew that I wouldn't be able to combine the two – my job involved frequent trips abroad. I could hardly travel with a baby in tow and at the same time I didn't want to leave my child with a stranger. My entire pregnancy was spent worrying about how I would cope. I became so depressed my work started to suffer before I'd even given birth.'

The most important thing for women to remember is that although it is possible to have it all, it is not always advisable to have it all at once. There is nothing wrong with taking a career break in order to have children, or indeed with returning to work straight after the birth. Every woman has different needs, but during pregnancy they are essentially the same – the need to stay calm and relaxed. This is what should influence your career decisions.

The growth in single-parent families

A growing number of women are having to face pregnancy and birth without a partner by their side. To cope with pregnancy as a single parent can be a very daunting experience. Jessica became pregnant as the result of a one-night stand. Here she recounts how her feelings changed during her pregnancy:

'When I first became pregnant I was actually very pleased, despite the fact that I wasn't in a relationship with the father. I have always been quite an insecure person and I felt that by having a child I would feel more complete – I would at last have somebody who would love me unconditionally. But after about three months I got so scared. I felt really lonely. Everywhere I went I seemed to see couples with their children – they always looked so happy. It got even worse when I started antenatal classes. All the other women brought their partners; I had to pair up with the midwife for my exercises. I felt like everybody was staring at me. In the end I started wishing that something terrible would happen to me – I could never have done anything to harm my baby, but I secretly hoped that something would go wrong. I wanted to die.'

All parents and all babies need to feel loved and secure and where this love and security stem from is not vitally important. Of course in an ideal world we would all live in our happy little units – mum, dad, baby and goldfish – with not a cross word uttered or a sullen look exchanged. However, we live in a world where one out of three marriages end in divorce and almost three out of three end in disappointment! There are millions of children growing up today in two-parent households where arguments and violence are a way of life. As a single parent you are just as capable of providing your child with love and support as any married couple. It is vital, however, that there is somebody there to give you love and support, whether it be a close friend or family member.

Financial problems

Financial problems are a well-known cause of distress and so it is hardly surprising that they should be linked to antenatal depression. Open any pregnancy magazine and you are confronted with countless glossy pictures of brightly painted nurseries, crammed full of expensive toys and beautifully carved furniture. It is guaranteed that you will never see a damp-ridden, cockroach-infested room on the nineteenth floor of an inner city tenement, a room bereft of toys and bright colours, with a makeshift cot and a second-hand mattress. But for many women beset with financial worries this is all they are able to provide for their new baby. Instead of being a time for excitedly decorating the nursery, pregnancy becomes a time for guilt and despair as women wonder how they will ever be able to provide for their unborn child. Sonia dreaded the arrival of her third child solely because of her financial difficulties:

'I didn't plan my third pregnancy – I was having enough trouble with my eldest two. My boyfriend Tony was out of work and we were barely making ends meet on his dole money and the little bit I earned from my part-time cleaning jobs. I had been on at the council for months and months about being re-housed – our flat was full of damp and both my kids were suffering from asthma. To make matters worse one of our neighbours was dealing drugs and all kinds of people would be walking past our flat morning, noon and night. I was smoking like a chimney and taking valium for my nerves and then I found out I was pregnant again. To be honest when I found out I just wanted to top myself. How could I bring another child into this? Some days when the other kids were at school I would pack a bag and sit on my bed trying to pluck up the courage to walk away from it all. I just wanted to walk out that door and never come back. No matter how hard I tried just couldn't find a way out of the mess I was in.'

If financial worries are casting a shadow over your pregnancy you really need to seek professional assistance. Are you getting all the benefits available to you? Have you looked at the different options open to you? Talking to somebody else about this, even if it is a friend rather than an official, can often help to uncover solutions you may never have thought of before.

Chapter 2
The Link Between Antenatal and Postnatal Depression and How to Break It

Although the majority of cases of antenatal depression disappear with the birth of the baby, in one-third of cases the mother will go on to suffer from postnatal depression, as the following examples demonstrate.

Mary

'After his birth the fears and anxieties immediately disappeared, but were gradually replaced by different feelings of concern and anxiety over my son. I felt quite lonely and vulnerable being alone with him and didn't know how to amuse him. My mind felt confused and miserable for about nine months after the birth.'

Bella

'I finally gave birth to a healthy, perfect and beautiful baby boy weighing 3.2kg (7lb 4oz). For the next couple of weeks I felt elated and even managed to realise that the way I had been throughout my pregnancy had been an over-reaction. However, at around three weeks after the birth I began to feel *bad about myself again. This time my thoughts revolved around whether it was fair to have had the baby at such a young age – I was 17. How could I possibly be a good mother? In the eyes of the law I wasn't even an adult. At my six-week check my GP diagnosed chronic postnatal depression. When I received the diagnosis something inside me snapped. Everything came pouring out. The doctor then told me that she suspected that as the depression before the birth had gone untreated this may have left me more susceptible to postnatal depression.'*

Recent studies have indeed supported Bella's doctor's diagnosis. In a 1997 review of postnatal depression written for perinatal health workers, V. N. Walther writes:

'When maternal anxiety and depression [during the pregnancy] are reduced, new-borns are also protected from the consequences of maternal deprivation which accompany postpartum depression.'[1]

This highlights the importance of treating antenatal depression in order to prevent postnatal depression for the sake of the child, as well as the mother.

How to Avoid Antenatal Depression Leading to Postnatal Depression

When I was heavily pregnant I remember reading in one of my many pregnancy books some tips on how to enjoy the first few weeks after the birth. The writer described how she and her husband would have picnics in bed with their new-born child, sipping glasses of wine and nibbling on cheese straws whilst listening to soothing music and watching their baby sleep. It all sounded idyllic and I longed to try it out for myself, but it was a complete disaster. Instead of soothing music the most common sounds in our bedroom those first few weeks were of the baby screaming followed by dad muttering, *'I'm sleeping in the spare room, some of us have got work in the morning!'* When I did get a few minutes' peace in bed the last thing I wanted to do was have a picnic – sleep was all I was interested in.

Looking back on it, I was completely unprepared for quite how tiring life with a new-born baby can be. I tried desperately to continue life as normal, struggling to learn the art of hoovering with a baby clamped to my breast, while simultaneously applying mascara and exercising my pelvic floor. And all on just two hours sleep! My friends commented on how well I was coping, but they didn't see me dissolving into an exhausted, tearful heap at the end of each day. If I had only taken the following simple steps towards the end of my pregnancy I would have had every chance of keeping postnatal depression at bay.

Dealing with antenatal depression

As Bella's experience proved, it is very important for sufferers of antenatal depression to face up to their feelings and try to deal with them before giving birth. The second part of this book looks into the ways in which to do this in far more detail, but perhaps the most beneficial thing you can do is to express how you are feeling. Whether this be to your doctor, midwife, a close friend or relative, try to get things off your chest. Counselling is probably the best way to do this as a counsellor is trained to give proper, constructive advice (see Chapter 6: Seeking Medical Help for further details).

Louisa found yoga particularly helpful in the last part of her pregnancy:

> *'Although my pregnancy had been planned, with hindsight I don't think I was really prepared for it. I became extremely depressed and was terrified of giving birth. I initially took up*

yoga in order to prepare for the birth physically, but it ended up helping me a great deal mentally as well. We were taught that the birth is a tremendous ordeal for the baby too and for the first time in my entire pregnancy I started to feel concern for my unborn child rather than just myself. I had been so wrapped up in my own fears I hadn't stopped to think about how frightening the birth process must be for a tiny baby. For the first time I felt a real maternal instinct towards my baby and I knew that I would have to be strong for his sake.'

This change in attitude late in Louisa's pregnancy probably played a vital role in her recovery from antenatal depression the instant her child was born, enabling her to bond with him straight away.

Coming to terms with becoming a parent

Becoming a parent is one of the main psychological causes of both antenatal and postnatal depression and is looked into in much more detail in the next chapter. This is particularly true for the first-time pregnancy, and the importance of the change in status and increased responsibility this involves cannot be underestimated. Becoming a parent can affect your relationships: with your partner, as any cracks suddenly become magnified; with your own parents, as you can be reminded of what was missing from your own childhood; and with your friends as socialising becomes increasingly difficult.

If you can come to terms with your change in status before the birth and realise all the positive aspects of becoming a parent it will go a long way towards avoiding problems once the child has arrived.

Ensure you have a comprehensive support network

To avoid the onset of postnatal depression it is essential that you have enough support in the days and weeks immediately following the birth. Support comes in many different forms, but can be broken down into the following five categories:

1. Emotional
Somebody you have a close, loving bond with, in whom you can trust and confide

2. Self-esteem
Somebody who acknowledges your skills and abilities, who will praise you and make you feel good about yourself

3. Practical
Somebody who will offer help with day-to-day chores such as cleaning, shopping, taking any other children to school

4. Educational
Somebody who can offer informative advice on parenting and childcare

5. Social
A group or activity you are involved with, bringing you into contact with like-minded people

In order to ensure that you have a fully comprehensive support network after the birth of your baby, complete the following simple exercise.

On a blank sheet of paper write the following five headings:

Emotional

Self-esteem

Practical

Educational

Social

Under each of these headings write the names of all the people who will be able to provide you with this type of support.

Here is an example to give you some ideas:

Emotional
Partner, best friend, sister, mother
Self-esteem
Work colleague or boss, younger relative or friend
Practical
Parents, mother-in-law, neighbour, friends, other mothers
Educational
Mother, more experienced parent, health visitor, doctor
Social
Church, political organisation, keep-fit class

If you find you seem to be lacking in support in any of these areas at least you have the time to try and do something about it before the baby arrives. Try talking to the people whose names you have written down before the birth and let them know how much you would appreciate their support. This is not a sign of weakness or inability to cope, it is just a matter of being practical. Why make your first few weeks with your new child a miserable experience if it really doesn't have to be? The people who care about you will be happy to help – just as you would be happy to help them in their hour of need.

Taking care of yourself

If you have been suffering from antenatal depression it will probably reach a peak by the last month of your pregnancy as your anxieties reach fever pitch and you become increasingly uncomfortable physically. Although you probably see little point in having a haircut or treating yourself to a facial this really is an ideal time to do so. A little bit of pampering could give your spirits a welcome lift, and it will be a while before you get the chance to do so once the baby arrives. (Remember of course to keep any new hairstyles practical – this is not really the best time for a high-maintenance hairdo!)

At the hospital

It is vital that you stay in hospital for as long a time (or in some cases, as short a time) as you need. If you had an exhausting overnight labour then try to stay in hospital until you feel rested. In hospital you only have to concentrate on your baby and yourself, rather than your husband and any other children. Alternatively, you may find hospital a very hard environment to relax in and long for the security of your own home. If this is the case discharge yourself as soon as is allowable. It is vital that those first few days with your baby are as stress-free as possible.

Returning home

The key thing to remember upon returning home is to avoid exhaustion at all costs. There is a tendency to admire women who give birth on a Monday and slip back into their size 8 clothes and high-powered career by Friday. But having a baby is a physically traumatic event and should be recognised as such: you would hardly go bouncing back into your previous life following major surgery and nor should you attempt to do so after giving birth. This is a once-in-a-lifetime chance to focus on bonding with your child so temporarily shelve the trivialities of life, such as polishing the budgie and cleaning out the cupboards. Don't worry if the house gets in a state – by avoiding feelings of guilt you may also prevent feelings of depression.

Keep a copy of the following checklist handy for when you bring your baby home and use it as your guide for the first few weeks:

Checklist for the first few weeks at home

Rest

Take every available opportunity to catch up on your sleep. You have the rest of your life to try and achieve the world's cleanest house, but for the next few weeks make sleep your number one priority.

Walk
As soon as you are able to, go out for walks. Fresh air, sunlight and getting out of the house will help you both physically and mentally.

Postnatal exercises
Begin your postnatal exercises as soon as possible, but avoid anything too strenuous for the first six weeks.

Get dressed
Try to avoid falling into the trap of still being in your dressing gown at tea time. Your own appearance should come before that of your house, so if it's a choice between shampooing your hair or the carpet, head for the shower.

Eat properly
There is a real danger of feeling too tired to eat anything but chocolate in these first few weeks. Lack of sleep tends to destroy the appetite but try to eat healthy snacks as well as sweets. (See Chapter Seven for more ideas on diet.) Invest in a good postnatal multivitamin and mineral supplement from your local chemist or health food shop.

Use your support network
Make full use of any offers of help and don't be afraid to ask.

Keep a diary
Not only of your baby's progress, but also your own. Use it to get any worries or fears off your chest. When you are feeling negative about something write about it – then re-read it and try to counter it with something positive that has happened that day.

Avoid unnecessary stress
This may seem like stating the obvious, but try to put off anything that you know will cause you additional stress, such as making major career decisions, moving house or getting divorced!

The Cases of Antenatal Depression that End With the Birth

It is important to remember that the majority of cases of antenatal depression end with the birth. So if you are suffering from ante-natal depression please do not think that this is a guaranteed passport to postnatal gloom. Two-thirds of sufferers experience instant and lasting relief the minute their child is born, as Louisa discovered:

'Straight after the birth Lee was taken to the nursery and I had a really good sleep. As soon as he was brought back to me I felt like it was Christmas. I stayed in hospital for five days and when I came home it felt almost as if I had been away in some kind of prison during my pregnancy and now I had finally been released. Everything seemed so much newer and brighter than it had been before and yet it was all exactly the same – it was me who had changed.'

Chapter 3
Postnatal Depression

What is Postnatal Depression?

It can never be said that postnatal depression is a recent development. As long ago as 400BC the Greek physician Hippocrates wrote about the existence of some form of depressive illness following childbirth in his third book of *Epidemics*. In the eighteenth century, a French doctor named Louis Marce wrote a paper on postnatal illness, but it was not until the 1960s that the first proper study was carried out. In 1968 Professor Brice Pitt studied the moods of 365 women during their pregnancy and after the birth. He found that 10 per cent of the women studied developed postnatal depression and this figure is still used as a benchmark today, although more recent studies suggest that the actual incidence of postnatal depression may be as high as 20 per cent.

As many as 90 per cent of new mothers experience some feelings of depression after the birth, usually emerging towards the end of the first two weeks. These can be broken down into three main categories:

- **The baby blues**
  The feelings of weepiness commonly associated with days 3–5 after the birth. It is experienced by 60–80 per cent of mothers and usually disappears after a few days.

- **Postnatal depression**
  Usually a gradual slide into depression following the birth, affecting about 10–20 per cent of mothers. It may start off as the

'baby blues' or it may begin to appear slightly later on. Most cases have gone within the first year of the birth.

- **Postpartum psychosis**
  This is by far the most serious psychiatric illness associated with childbirth, affecting one mother in 1,000. It usually occurs within the first two weeks of the birth, often in women with a history of manic depression, when without warning the mother becomes psychotic. The symptoms are far more severe than the weepiness of the 'baby blues'. From extreme paranoia to hearing voices and losing a grip on reality, postpartum psychosis is a terrifying experience for the sufferer. However, once diagnosed there is a range of treatments available and there is no reason for the sufferer not to make a full recovery.

The reality of postnatal depression

As with antenatal depression, the sufferer of postnatal depression experiences a range of feelings that are completely contrary to those commonly associated with becoming a new mother, as the following stories show.

Jennifer's story

'I loved every minute of my pregnancy. I had no problems with morning sickness, I had tons of energy – I carried on exercising right up until the birth – and I was very excited at the prospect of having my first child. Although my labour was extremely long – almost 24 hours in total – I finally gave birth to a healthy baby boy with no major complications. I was completely shattered, however, and for some reason I found it impossible to feel any excitement once he arrived. All I wanted to do was go to sleep. My husband was ecstatic and all he could talk about was how happy he was. He's not normally an emotional man and yet he was crying his eyes out, whereas I didn't feel a thing, only tired.

'I had been up for two days and yet I just didn't seem able to get to sleep. I was terrified that if I did my baby might stop breathing. So I lay there watching him all night. The next day I returned home thinking that once I was back in my normal surroundings things would improve, but if anything things just got worse. I couldn't seem to bond with my son and yet I was paranoid about his safety. Everything had to be sterilised, I would force myself to stay awake so that I could watch him breathing and I was absolutely terrified of cot death syndrome. When the midwife or health visitor came to see me I made out that everything was fine – I was far too ashamed to admit the truth – that I couldn't cope. As the weeks went on things just got worse and worse. Housework seemed impossible and then I'd sit there in my messy house, that had always been so spotless before, and feel even more of a failure. I lost all my self-respect; I didn't care about my own appearance any more; I didn't care about life to be honest. Some nights I would go and sit in the bathroom and hold a razor in my hand trying to summon up the courage to end it all. On other occasions I wished I could just go to sleep for a long, long time and when I finally woke up everything would be back to how it used to be, before I ever got pregnant.

'One night my husband found me in the bathroom and realised what I was thinking of doing. The next day he made me an emergency appointment with my GP and that was the turning point for me. As soon as she diagnosed postnatal depression it was as if a huge cloud started to lift. I was put on Prozac and went to regular counselling sessions for about three months. As I talked through all my feelings with my counsellor I started to feel love for my baby for the first time. And as I got better this love grew stronger and stronger.

'My son is now two years old, I am no longer on medication and I don't need the counselling any more. Things are back to normal, but I will always feel guilty about how I was *those first few months, and I do worry about any long-term effect it may have had on my son.'*

Olivia's story

'I suffered from postnatal depression for about seven months after the birth of my youngest child. The pregnancy hadn't been planned and I don't know if that had anything to do with it, but from the moment I got home it wasn't like with the other two – I just felt no enjoyment in having a new baby. I was resentful that I was stuck at home all day and I didn't see the point in making an effort any more. I suppose I felt worthless. I had no patience with my baby when she cried. I felt I was too old and too tired to be running around after a new baby. I started to hate my husband and couldn't stand him even sleeping in the same bed as me. Then I would worry myself sick that he would start having an affair.

'One day when my daughter just wouldn't stop crying I started screaming and screaming at her to be quiet. In the end I had to leave the room as I was so scared I was going to hurt her. That is when I realised I needed help. I rang the Association for Postnatal Illness and ended up speaking to a wonderful woman who had actually experienced postnatal depression herself. Through talking to her I realised I was not alone in what I was going through. I ended up having weekly therapy and as I started to address my problems I became overwhelmed with feelings of guilt. I had been completely selfish and will always regret the fact that my daughter never received the love she deserved in those first few months.'

The Pressures Facing a New Mother

Along with her bundle of joy, the mother of a new-born baby also brings home a bundle of pressures, all of which, if unprepared, can trigger feelings of hopelessness and despair. The current crop of celebrity mums with their seemingly elastic abdominals and their cleverly applied make-up give the impression that it is all a breeze, but who knows what goes on when the cameras aren't around? In fact, in recent years many other celebrity mums have come forward to talk of their own experiences of postnatal depression, proving that no amount of money or privileges can fully protect a new mother from the following pressures of parenthood:

- Lack of sleep leading to feelings of exhaustion
- Being on call to a baby 24 hours a day
- A need to be constantly vigilant regarding the baby's health and well-being
- Physical pain or discomfort from the after-effects of the birth
- Lack of any kind of routine
- Loss of freedom; the sense of being house-bound
- Potential difficulties with breast-feeding
- Stress upon relationship with partner.

The good news is that all these pressures should start to diminish after about six weeks. Your baby will start to sleep for longer periods of time at night, any physical side effects from the birth, such as stitches, will hopefully have disappeared, feeding will become easier as you become more accustomed to it, you will be able to return to some kind of routine in your life and, most importantly, you will start to feel your old self once more. It is absolutely crucial that you keep this in mind during those first few weeks as a glimmer of light at the end of the tunnel. It is all too easy to fall into the trap of believing that things will never return to normal, and this is when feelings of despair can quickly lead to feelings of depression.

What is Wrong With Me?

If you have given birth recently and are feeling low it may help to compare your own symptoms with those listed below in order to identify exactly the form of depression from which you are suffering.

Symptoms of the 'baby blues'

- **Physical** – Lack of sleep, loss of appetite, constantly lethargic
- **Mental** – Anxiety, nervousness, over-emotional, lack of confidence, negative about physical appearance, sorrow, feeling out of your depth, confused
- **Behaviour** – Tearful, over-sensitive, hyperactive, lack of feeling for your baby.

If, three or four days after the birth, you suddenly find yourself in floods of tears it is quite likely to be a case of the 'baby blues'. As the initial euphoria dies down doubts and fears may start to creep in. 'Why haven't I bonded with my baby?' 'How will I cope with this new responsibility?' 'Will I ever be my old self again?' These are all quite natural worries and may cause you to feel weepy for the next couple of days. After the excitement of giving birth to her first child, Susan suddenly found herself unable to stop crying:

'I'd finally given birth to my son Jake at half past nine in the morning, following an exhausting 14-hour labour. Almost immediately we were taken up to the maternity ward where we were besieged by friends and family, and this continued all day. By the evening when I was finally alone with my baby I felt completely shattered. I lay there on my own in that ward looking at this little bundle in the cot beside me and suddenly I felt terrified. All the excitement of the day disappeared and I was left feeling scared and depressed. Even though I was exhausted I couldn't get to sleep and I spent most of the night wandering up and down the ward. I was worried that I wouldn't be able to cope – I had never changed a nappy or bathed a baby in my life – I didn't have a clue how I was going to manage. For the next couple of days in hospital I felt as if I had a split personality – happy and cheery in front of the doctors and visitors and in floods of tears whenever I was alone. I felt as if I had become a different person overnight, that I was having some kind of breakdown, but when I got

back home everything seemed to fall into place. Every day my confidence grew and by the time my baby was a couple of weeks old I was back to my old self again.'

Symptoms of postnatal depression

If you have recently given birth and feel that things seem to be getting steadily worse rather than better, and you find yourself experiencing any of the following symptoms, you may well be suffering from postnatal depression.

- **Physical** – Headaches, dizziness, tingling feeling in limbs, chest pains, heart palpitations, hyperventilating, feelings of faintness, loss of interest in sex
- **Mental** – Despair, inability to cope, feelings of inadequacy, chronic anxiety (especially over the baby's health), lack of concentration, apathy, suicidal tendencies, bizarre thoughts
- **Behaviour** – Panic attacks, hostility, inability to bond with the baby, aggressive tendencies, phobias, nightmares, extreme guilt, fear for own sanity.

Jane had a problem-free pregnancy with her second child, but after a difficult labour she found it impossible to bond with her baby:

'It's quite ironic that I had a far better pregnancy with my second child than with my first – I felt great and had loads of energy throughout – and yet I went on to develop postnatal depression. Because I had had no problems with the birth of my first child I was completely relaxed when I went into labour for the second time. However, after a few hours I had to have an emergency caesarean because my baby was in a non-engaged breech position. I was absolutely terrified at the time but everything went smoothly and I gave birth to a healthy baby girl. After the birth I was taken up to the ward and from that moment on I just couldn't stop crying. I was so tired and in so much pain I couldn't even get out of bed to

pick up my baby when she needed feeding. I had to wait for the midwife to bring her to me which made me feel totally useless. When I got home things got steadily worse. All I wanted to do was stay in bed all day, I had no energy and I started to really resent both of my children. I would have panic attacks at the slightest thing. I would feel dizzy and faint and sometimes I would feel as if I couldn't breathe. I couldn't bear the sound of my baby crying and my eldest child, who had just turned three, really suffered because I was on such a short fuse all the time. I became convinced that I wasn't cut out to be a mother and I seriously thought that it was only a matter of time before my kids were taken into care. Eventually I became so scared I might lose control completely that I went to see my GP. It had taken me four months to become desperate enough to seek help. I was so ashamed of the feelings I was having – it was only when I thought my children might be in danger that I actually plucked up the courage to do something. I only wish that I had done it sooner. My doctor was very understanding and supportive. He immediately diagnosed chronic postnatal depression and prescribed antidepressants. I was very wary of taking any kind of medication; I didn't want to end up hooked on anything, but I also knew that I couldn't carry on the way I was going. Slowly but surely the antidepressants began to lift me. I'd start having the odd good day here and there and gradually the good days became more frequent. My daughter was a year old when I finally came off the antidepressants. It's been a long hard slog, but I finally feel as if I am returning to my old self. I still have the odd day where I doubt my ability as a mother and I feel incredibly guilty for what I put my kids through, but on the whole life is good once more and I can look forward to the future with a bit more confidence.'

As with antenatal depression, sufferers of postnatal depression are left feeling isolated and confused. Instead of enjoying the experience of parenthood it becomes an uphill struggle fraught with problems, feelings of guilt and inadequacy, and all for no apparent reason. There are, however, a wide range of potential causes of postnatal depression that need to be examined in close detail in order to achieve a better understanding of this illness.

Symptoms of postpartum psychosis

- **Physical** – Frantic over-activity, refusal to eat, loss of need to sleep
- **Mental** – Extreme confusion, bizarre hallucinations, loss of memory, incoherence, very fast thoughts and speech, delusions, feelings of paranoia, hearing voices
- **Behaviour** – Suspiciousness, irrational statements or actions, easily distracted, restless.

If you suspect that you may be suffering from postpartum psychosis you must immediately seek help from your doctor as this can be a very dangerous illness if left untreated. The good news is that, once diagnosed, you have every chance of making a total recovery and enjoying your role as a mother to the full, as the following example demonstrates:

Cindy had no history of any kind of mental illness prior to the birth of her son and yet a week after he was born she became psychotic, experiencing extreme paranoid delusions:

'From the moment my son was born I didn't feel quite right – my husband said I was acting all spaced out – but we put it down to tiredness. However, by about six or seven days after the birth I started to have really strange thoughts. I didn't think that they were strange at the time. I became convinced that my whole family were out to get me and that they were planning to harm me and my baby in some way. The only person I trusted was my husband, but after a couple of weeks I even began to doubt him. As soon as he went to work I would search through his things for some

*kind of clue that he was part of the conspiracy. I became
convinced that our flat was bugged and would spend the
whole day pushing my son around in his pram – I thought
we were safer outside. I would walk for miles with my mind
racing. Who was involved? Had that stranger sitting on the
bench been sent to spy on me? How was I going to escape?
At first I pretended everything was fine because I didn't
want to let my family know I was on to them, but as I
became more and more terrified for my safety I refused to
see anybody. Finally my husband called the doctor out to see
me. Of course I thought that she was part of the conspiracy
too, but she finally convinced me to come with her to the
hospital. I ended up being hospitalised for almost six weeks,
but my baby was allowed to stay with me in a specialist
mother and baby unit. After about four weeks the medication I was on started to take effect and I gradually returned
to the real world. I was absolutely horrified by what had
happened to me, the things I had accused my family of and
the stress I had caused my husband. I had to be treated for
depression for quite some time afterwards, but slowly I
picked up the pieces and started all over again. My son is
now three years old. I am off the medication and I am feeling happier than I have done in a long time. I don't think I
will ever have another child though, and that is something
that saddens me a great deal as I always dreamed of having
a large family, but I could never put myself or my family
through that again.'*

Although postpartum psychosis can be part of a long-term
recurring problem, with some sufferers remaining on medication
for life, in the majority of cases it is relatively easy to treat once
diagnosed. Unfortunately once it has occured there is an increased
risk of it happening in subsequent pregnancies, and owing to the
traumatic nature of the illness, many sufferers are left extremely
reluctant to have another child.

The Causes of Postnatal Depression

Physical causes

Hormonal

During pregnancy the levels of the hormone progesterone in the mother increase by between 50 and 100 times, and yet within three days of giving birth they will be back to their normal, pre-pregnancy level. For years this dramatic drop has been considered one of the most significant factors behind postnatal depression. A study of 27 new mothers carried out in 1976 found that those women with the greatest levels of depression also experienced the greatest drop in progesterone.[1] Dr Katharina Dalton, one of the first doctors to study and treat postnatal depression also came to the same conclusion, pioneering the use of progesterone suppositories or injections as a treatment. Oestrogen is another hormone that falls sharply after the birth of a baby and one study has shown that oestrogen patches can prove effective in the treatment of postnatal depression.

Although there is some evidence that such a drastic drop in hormone levels can be linked to the baby blues, current research is moving away from the link with postnatal depression. A study carried out in 1996 argues that there is, *'no support for a direct association of progesterone with postnatal mood at six weeks post-partum'*.[2]

While it makes sense that the fall in progesterone and oestrogen levels will affect the mood of some women, more research is definitely required and, as with antenatal depression, there are many other factors, physical, emotional and social, that need to be taken into account.

Premenstrual syndrome

There is no evidence to suggest that sufferers of premenstrual syndrome are any more likely to suffer from postnatal depression. However, there is some evidence to suggest that sufferers of postnatal depression will go on to suffer from PMS. Dr Dalton found that as many as 90 per cent of sufferers of postnatal depression who had never suffered from PMS previously would go on to develop it as their depression faded. It appears that this is all part of a gradual process of recovery, as in most cases the PMS also improved with time.

Thyroid problems

The thyroid gland produces the hormones responsible for controlling our metabolism, energy levels and body temperature. Immediately after pregnancy the levels of these hormones drop and in a about 6–7 per cent of women this can lead to a condition known as hypothyroidism (an underactive thyroid gland). The symptoms of hypothyroidism are very similar to those of postnatal depression and therefore sufferers can be wrongly diagnosed. Hypothyroidism causes lack of energy, weight gain for no apparent reason, constipation and feelings of despair. If you suspect you may be suffering from an underactive thyroid a simple blood test from your GP will be able to put your mind at rest. If hypothyroidism is diagnosed it is easily treated with hormone replacement medication and the symptoms should disappear within a matter of weeks. Thyroid hormone levels should return to normal within six months.

Anaemia

An illness commonly confused with postnatal depression, owing to it's similar symptoms, is anaemia. During pregnancy a woman's iron stores become depleted and this can worsen if a lot of blood is lost during the labour. As with thyroid problems a simple blood test can ascertain whether or not you are suffering from anaemia and it is easily treated with high-dosage iron supplements and an iron-rich diet.

Breast-feeding

Breast-feeding can be linked to feelings of depression in two ways. First, a huge emphasis is placed upon the importance of breast-feeding. Mothers are taught that breast-feeding is the 'natural' way; books and magazines are full of pictures of women gazing contentedly at the baby sucking eagerly at their breast. They never print pictures of the tear-streaked faces of mothers trying to pacify hysterical babies unable to latch on to excruciatingly sore nipples. Breast-feeding can be a soul-destroying experience for some women, made all the worse by their feelings of having somehow failed as a mother. Yvonne had been looking forward to breast-feeding her first baby, but found that it was not at all as she expected:

'I put my postnatal depression down to the problems I had with breast-feeding. Admittedly tiredness also played a large part, but it was the disappointment at not being able to feed my daughter that made me feel like a total failure for several months. At first I just couldn't seem to do it right. No matter what position I held my baby in she didn't seem able to latch on to my nipple. I would become frantic and so would she and we'd both sit there wailing. After a few days it did start to get a bit easier but I found it very uncomfortable; my nipples were sore and my breasts would get so swollen and painful. I started dreading feeds, they almost felt like a battleground – I can't explain it really. I just hated the whole experience and that made me hate myself. My husband suggested that we start using formula milk and I'll never forget the first time he gave her a bottle. I sat there watching them together and I felt a complete failure. What kind of mother was I that I couldn't even feed my baby properly? And of course there were all the health worries. Everywhere I would read about the benefits of breast-feeding and yet I wasn't able to give my daughter what was best for her. When she was four weeks old I had completely stopped breast-feeding and for the next couple of months I felt incredibly guilty and depressed. I felt as if I hadn't bonded properly with my baby and I'm sure that was due to the fact that there had been so much stress between us so early on. I was jealous of the love that my husband felt for

her – why couldn't I feel the same way? Slowly but surely things got better. My baby seemed perfectly healthy on the formula milk and I became a lot more relaxed. I would say it took me about four months before I had completely bonded with her – it was a slow, gradual process – but once it came my feelings of depression and failure disappeared.'

There is no doubt that breast milk is better for a baby than formula milk. However, there is also no doubt that a relaxed, happy mother is far better for a baby than a stressed-out wreck. If at all possible, it is well worth sticking with breast-feeding for at least the first three days as this is when the breasts produce colostrum. This is a light, yellow-coloured liquid that contains valuable antibodies from the mother's immune system which will protect her baby from illnesses such as polio and influenza. The chances are that by the end of three days any initial problems with feeding will have disappeared, but if not try using the following techniques:

Overcoming breast-feeding difficulties

- Make your environment as comfortable as possible. Use cushions or pillows to get into the best position for you and the baby.
- Relax; watch TV or read a magazine, have a drink or snack yourself while feeding.
- Sit up straight and hold the baby up towards you rather than leaning over to her. This removes pressure from your back and shoulders.
- Use a pump to remove excess milk if your breasts become swollen and hard.
- Expressed milk can also be used in a bottle to give you a break from feeding.
- If a nipple becomes unbearably sore express from that breast and only let the baby feed from the other one.
- If you start to feel feverish and your breast becomes red consult your doctor, as you could be suffering from a blocked duct.

If all this fails and you find breast-feeding is causing distress to you and your baby then you must make a positive decision to move to formula milk. It is important not to view this as a sign of failure, but rather an attempt to provide your baby with a happy, stress-free environment.

Positive reasons for bottle feeding

- If you have managed to breast-feed for the first three days you will have given your baby the best possible start in life.
- Millions of children have been bottle fed with no ill-effects.
- A baby needs a happy, relaxed mother.
- By eliminating a source of stress between yourself and your baby you will find it easier to bond and develop a loving relationship.

Weaning

Another possible connection between breast-feeding and postnatal depression is weaning and the hormonal changes it involves. As soon as you stop breast-feeding, the level of the hormone prolactin drops. Many women report feeling weepy and low around the time of weaning and if this is combined with any feelings of guilt or failure then depression can follow.

Complications with the birth

Complications during the birth can be a terrifying experience and in some cases it can take several months for the mother to recover. One British study of postnatal depression found that as many as 55 per cent of the sufferers studied had had some kind of obstetric intervention during the birth. With the immediate arrival of a new baby and all the work it involves there is little time for a woman to come to terms with the fear she experienced. This can later manifest itself in feelings of depression and can lead to difficulties bonding with the baby as the following women found.

Everything was going smoothly during the birth of Abbey's first child when suddenly her cervix stopped dilating.

'My baby was facing the wrong way and had somehow got stuck and I was told that I would have to have some kind of hormone drip which would make my contractions far more violent. I had managed up to this point with no pain relief, but I decided that if it was going to get worse I ought to have something, so I opted for a Pethidine injection. I went from feeling completely in control of my labour to completely out of control. I felt as if my body had been taken over and the drugs made me totally spaced out. I can't even remember the moment my son was born. I just had no interest – I didn't even ask what sex he was or if he was okay – I just felt completely traumatised. For days afterwards I felt dazed and I can honestly say, although it breaks my heart to do so, I felt no love for my baby. I was so out of it when he arrived they might just as well have brought him from somewhere else. It didn't feel as if he had come from inside me. I had to ask my husband to describe every detail of his arrival over and over again, but it made no difference, it felt as if I wasn't even there. As the weeks went by this little baby was like a stranger to me and I felt as if I was going mad. How could I not love my own child, my only child? I became extremely depressed and I honestly thought that I would never be able to love him properly. When I read about the special bond that exists between a mother and her son I felt completely inadequate and useless.'

Margaret blames her emergency caesarean for her postnatal depression:

'I had been very nervous about giving birth throughout my pregnancy and when they told me at the last minute that I was going to need an emergency caesarean I was absolutely terrified. I truly believed that I was going to die and I remember wishing that I'd never got pregnant. Even when it all went smoothly and I gave birth to a healthy baby boy I felt *totally numb inside. I didn't feel any excitement or euphoria. Perhaps it was the physical side-effects of the caesarean, the discomfort and the exhaustion, but I had no enthusiasm for anything any more – not for my baby, not for my husband, not for myself. I didn't bother getting dressed or going out, I didn't see the point in anything. I would never have harmed my baby and I always made sure he was properly looked after, but it was as if I was on autopilot. I think subconsciously I was blaming him for putting me through the trauma in the hospital.'*

Both cases highlight the need for some kind of counselling immediately after a traumatic birth in order to avoid the initial feelings of fear and confusion developing into long-term depression later on.

Previous infertility

Ironically, previous problems with infertility can be linked to post-natal depression. A significant number of women who have become pregnant as a result of IVF treatment after years of trying, subsequently fall victim to postnatal depression. Many women spend years trying to get pregnant and over the course of those years their whole lives can start to revolve around this unfulfilled dream. The more disappointments they have the more attractive the idea of having a baby becomes. Pregnancy becomes the answer to all their problems and heartache, but when it finally arrives there is always the danger that the reality won't match the dream.

Lucy finally became pregnant after 12 years of trying and her third attempt at IVF:

'From the moment we got married Dave and I were desperate to start a family, but it never happened. Every month I would ride this roller-coaster: excitement building up towards

the end of the month – followed by total devastation every time my period started. It got worse and worse over the years and we would take our disappointment out on each other. We even split up twice, but we always came back together. Eventually we made the decision to go for IVF and finally I became pregnant. I can't begin to describe how excited we were, but I also spent most of my pregnancy terrified that something would go wrong and I would lose the baby – I had had so many set-backs I couldn't believe that we were finally going to have a child of our own. But we did and I gave birth to a healthy baby girl. The first couple of weeks were amazing – the moment we had dreamed of for all those years had finally arrived. At first I didn't mind the sleepless nights, I felt so lucky to have her, but I just seemed to get tireder and tireder as the weeks went on. I resented the fact that Dave could go off to work and continue his life as normal whereas I had all the night feeds and lack of sleep to contend with. I started to let things slip, like the cleaning and my own appearance. Suddenly I was back to all the old feelings, but this time instead of feeling depressed because I could not get pregnant I was depressed because I could not be a good mother. Once again I felt like a total failure.'

The pressures of having a new-born baby can be magnified if it has been your life's dream for so long. Years spent imagining how perfect those first few weeks would be can make the reality a total shock to the system. It is vital to remember that parenthood, like infertility, has its own sets of stresses and strains.

Physical problems following the birth

There are a number of physical problems following the birth that can cause great discomfort to the mother. Combined with exhaustion and all the other pressures of life with a new-born baby it can often lead to feelings of hopelessness and despair.

Episiotomy

An episiotomy is an incision made in the perineum in order to aid delivery of the baby. It is usually carried out if the baby's head is proving too large for normal delivery, if the foetus is in some kind of distress or if the baby is in a breech position. After the birth the incision is stitched back up. Most stitches dissolve after five or six days but the discomfort of the bruising may linger on. This discomfort can lead to other problems such as difficulties with breast-feeding or going to the toilet, but there are steps you can take to ease the problem:

- Bath in salt water to speed up the healing process.
- Use an inflatable rubber ring to sit on, especially when breast-feeding.
- Avoid constipation by eating a diet high in fibre.

There can be nothing more depressing than discovering that the pain does not actually end with the birth. Pain coupled with exhaustion can be a lethal combination but, as with all of the additional pressures of having a new baby, everything gets easier with time. Stitches dissolve and scars heal and before you know it you will be able to sit down without a care in the world once more.

Inability to lose weight

Already identified as a contributory factor to antenatal depression, excessive weight gain can also play a large part in postnatal depression. It can be hugely disappointing to give birth to a baby and yet still look as if you are heavily pregnant, but for many women this is what happens. It is all very well for celebrity mums to turn up for the obligatory photo shoot two weeks after giving birth, poured into a pair of size 8 jeans and a boob tube, but most of us are not fortunate enough to have the support of an army of personal fitness trainers, nutritionists, nannies and astrologers. Preparing a nutritious meal or performing 200 sit-ups are probably the last things on earth you feel like doing when dealing with the demands of a new-born baby on your own. It is enough just to drag yourself from the sofa to the next cup of coffee and chocolate bar and so, fuelled by lack of sleep, a cycle of inactivity, poor diet and depression begins.

Tracey's story

'At one of my last antenatal classes a woman came to talk to us about the recent birth of her child. She was incredibly slim and when somebody asked her about her weight she cheerily announced that the minute she gave birth she was back wearing her old jeans – the weight had literally dropped off her. This really cheered me up as I hadn't put too much weight on myself – it seemed to be all baby. However, when I gave birth I was so disappointed. I still had a huge pot belly and my breasts seemed to sag almost down to my waist! I was so depressed at still having to wear maternity clothes and yet I couldn't seem to get motivated to do any exercise. I was tired all the time and although I knew I shouldn't, I ate sweets continuously. Every time I had to feed my baby I would sit there munching my way through a box of chocolates or a bag of sweets. It started off as a way of getting energy, but soon I was comfort eating. I felt depressed because of my size and this made me eat even more. I felt guilty and resentful and although I loved my baby to bits I had no enthusiasm for anything any more. It took all my energy to keep her washed and dressed and fed – I let myself and my house go completely. I can honestly say it was one of the lowest points in my life and yet it should have been one of the happiest.'

Sufferers of all forms of depression often find themselves seeking comfort in the wrong type of foods. For women who are already concerned about their weight this can be a recipe for disaster as a cycle of guilt and despair is soon created. Breaking this cycle is undoubtedly tough, but adopting a healthier diet and lifestyle can often be the first steps out of depression.

The Emotional Causes of Postnatal Depression

Becoming a parent and the effects upon your existing relationships

With your mother

No matter how old, experienced or successful you are, becoming a parent can bring a child-like vulnerability to the strongest of women. As you prepare to become a mother yourself there is a natural tendency to re-examine your relationship with your own mother. If that relationship is a positive, loving and supportive one you will feel a sense of security and confidence in the challenges that lie ahead. If, however, your relationship is troubled, or you are indeed estranged, any unresolved conflicts can suddenly come back to haunt you and can be linked to both antenatal and postnatal depression.

Natalie spent her entire childhood playing an almost parental role to her alcoholic mother. As well as drinking heavily her mother was also prone to severe bouts of depression.

> *'I remember quite clearly one incident when I was 12 years old, where I had to talk my mother out of killing herself. I was terrified of leaving her to go to school – every day I would run home praying that I wouldn't find her dead. Of course I never did; she'd just be sitting there drunk and feeling sorry for herself as usual.'*

Natalie left home at 18 to go to university and never returned home.

> *'I just put it all behind me and threw myself into my work. I worked all the hours God sent setting up my own business, I married a kind and supportive man and I thought I had put all of the past behind me.'*

But this was not the case. When she became pregnant last year at the age of 32, Natalie's childhood experiences all came flooding back.

> *'I was reading a pregnancy magazine and a woman was talking about how her mother had moved in with her and her husband for the first two weeks after their baby was born. She was saying she didn't know how she would have coped without her mother there to do the cooking and cleaning and generally help her with the new baby. I suddenly felt this huge surge of anger at my own mother for not being there to help me. For the rest of my pregnancy and the first few months after my baby was born it was as if I relived every moment of my childhood. If I was not crying I was screaming and shouting – at my husband mainly, but sometimes I even shouted at my baby. This made me feel even worse because I thought I was going to turn out just as bad a mother as she was.'*

There are many different circumstances that can trigger feelings such as these. If your mother lives a long way away or if she died when you were still a child, these facts can trigger depression either during pregnancy or immediately afterwards. By trying to be a good mother to your own child you are made painfully aware of what you yourself missed out on. Feelings of resentment towards your mother can subconsciously be directed towards your baby as you swing between the desire to give your own child everything you were denied and anger at all you had to go without. If you believe your relationship with your mother is at the root of your antenatal or postnatal depression you must confront the problem head on. If it is impossible to talk to your mother herself speak to a friend, partner or counsellor.

With your partner

It is easy to imagine that the arrival of a new child will bring nothing but happiness and strength to the relationship of the parents.

But in those first few weeks of sleepless nights, dirty nappies and permanent exhaustion, tempers become frayed and marriages often become battlegrounds fraught with resentment and hostility. Possible sources of tension are as follows:

- Lack of sleep making both partners irritable and over-sensitive
- Sex or even the most basic signs of affection such as a cuddle go out of the window as sleep becomes the number one priority
- Mother only has enough energy for her baby, leaving father feeling left out
- Mother resents father for being able to escape to work
- Father resents mother for being able to stay at home all day
- Both partners experience a lack of understanding from the other
- Mother becomes convinced that partner will be tempted into an affair
- Father feels jealous of the love and affection the baby receives from the mother

These are just some of the potential trouble spots that follow the birth of a child. The euphoria and sense of togetherness experienced in the hospital can soon give way to shouting, sulking and the slamming of doors, as Moira and Paul soon discovered.

Moira's story

'We were overjoyed when Rachel was born as we had been trying to conceive for several years. Paul and I were very happily married and it didn't dawn on me for a moment that having a child would cause so many problems for us. Paul had two weeks off work after I had Rachel and it was lovely. We spent most of the time just the three of us together, our own little family. It was when Paul went back to work that everything started to go wrong. When he suggested that he sleep in the living room so that he could get a good night's sleep I was really upset. I remember getting up for the 2am feed and thinking of him sleeping soundly downstairs and I would feel *a mixture of jealousy and resentment. It was the same during the day. I would be up to my eyes in housework and dirty nappies and I would picture him laughing and joking with his friends in the office and going to the pub at lunchtime. It seemed so unfair that we were both Rachel's parents and yet I was the one who had to do all the work, I was the one who had to get up night after night. As I got more depressed and resentful I just shut Paul out. I didn't want him near me. I didn't want to hear his tales about work and his friends. I would look in the mirror and see this wreck staring back at me and I blamed Paul for ruining my life. One day Paul finally snapped and asked me if I wanted him to leave. I was so shocked that it had come to this, it made me realise that however bad it had got I didn't want a divorce. We started going to marriage guidance counselling and it was as if we had to learn to communicate all over again. Paul said a lot of things in the counselling sessions that I had no idea he was feeling and I started to realise how much he was going through too.'*

Paul's story

'I was so proud of Moira when she gave birth to Rachel and how she seemed to take to motherhood so naturally. When I went back to work I felt a bit jealous – we had spent two weeks together and now I felt a bit left out. When I got home at night I would watch Moira feeding Rachel and I realised that there was this bond between them that didn't include me. I was also going through a tough time at work. I had a very poor relationship with my boss and I really wanted to leave, but obviously we had just had a new baby and I didn't want to do anything to jeopardise our financial security. As the months went by Moira seemed to hate me more and more and I couldn't understand why. She seemed to have no interest in anything other than Rachel. I felt totally unwanted and in the

end I gave her an ultimatum – either we sort out our problems or we might as well get divorced. Of course I didn't want us to split up, but I felt desperate – the situation at home had become completely unbearable.'

The pressures of having a new baby are not just confined to the mother as this example clearly shows. Fathers have to contend with their own additional stresses and responsibilities. The danger is that both partners think they are the only one under any kind of pressure. Rather than talking to each other, a barrier of bitterness and resentment is built up which becomes increasingly difficult to break down. Relationship problems can obviously be linked to depression. For sufferers of postnatal depression this creates a cycle of despair: as your relationship crumbles you feel increasingly hopeless; as you feel increasingly hopeless you make less of an effort with your relationship. The only way to break this cycle is by honest and open communication, preferably with an objective mediator such as a marriage guidance counsellor or a close, neutral friend or relative.

The unsupportive or abusive partner

The strains of having a new child become even harder to bear if your partner is unsupportive or abusive. In those first few weeks after the birth your partner plays a vital role in your support network. Having another adult to share some of the burden of the late night feeds, nappy changing and housework can make a world of difference. However, if that support is not forthcoming it is all too easy for the mother to feel overwhelmed by the enormity of events, as Linda soon discovered:

'When I was pregnant I hadn't minded Chris playing foot- ball with his friends at all. I was still able to go out shopping with my friends and do my own thing. However, once I gave birth it was as if my life was put on hold whereas he expected to continue as normal – working all week then out playing

football at the weekend. When I asked him to stay at home with us at the weekend he became quite annoyed and said that football was his only way to unwind after the stresses of a week at work. He seemed to think that because I was at home all day I didn't need any sort of release. He also used that as a reason not to help with anything around the house. He said I was the one at home all day so I had plenty of time to get the housework done and look after our baby. He wouldn't even help with the washing up and I don't think he ever once bathed our son or changed a nappy. He carried on going out drinking after work as well – some nights not getting back until after closing time. I felt completely isolated and I'm sure that was behind my depression. It was as if I no longer had a life and I was forced to watch everybody else getting on with theirs.'

If your partner is being unsupportive you must confront the problem head on rather than build up a wall of silence and resentment between you. Rather than screaming and shouting (however tempting this may be) try to communicate your feelings in a constructive manner and, if all else fails, appeal to his sense of self-interest. For example:

'If you were to help out more with the feeds / doing the dishes / preparing the tea darling, I wouldn't be nearly so tired and I'd have far more time for you and your scintillating views on the off-side trap!'

If you are being abused by your partner then you must seek help, for your baby's sake as well as your own. If you are unable to turn to friends or family members then contact a women's group such as Refuge for advice and support. You must never suffer in silence.

With your friends

As with antenatal depression, your relationship with your friends can be a significant factor in postnatal depression. This is particularly true if those friends do not have children themselves. They may not appreciate the pressures you are under and may not understand any changes in you. Sarah lost one of her closest friends shortly after the birth of her first child.

> 'I was feeling a bit low – I think it was probably a case of the baby blues – and I really didn't want to see anybody. I just wanted to be alone with my son and recover from the birth and try and catch up on my sleep. One of my friends became really funny with me when I asked her not to come around. We used to see each other practically every day before. I think she felt that I didn't want to know her now I had my baby, but it wasn't like that at all – I just wanted some rest. I then found out that she had been criticising me to other friends and I was devastated. Normally I would have rung her up and had it out with her, but I was feeling so down and exhausted anyway I just crumpled. I cried for days – I completely over-reacted, with hindsight – but at the time all I could think about was how little she must have thought of me. Our whole friendship suddenly seemed a sham. I was depressed for about three months before I finally asked my GP for help. She wanted to prescribe antidepressants, but I was too scared of becoming addicted to medication so I went to see a therapist a few times which I found very helpful. By the time I was back to normal, too much time had passed and our friendship was beyond saving. I still feel angry that she reacted so childishly and put me through so much at such a vulnerable time in my life.'

Friends are an essential part of a new mother's support network, particularly during the day when your partner is probably at work, leaving you alone with your baby for long periods of time. True friends will appreciate the fact that you need time to get back on your feet following the birth. It is a very good idea to try and make new friends with women in similar situations so that you can provide support for each other. See your GP or health visitor for details of local mother and baby groups.

Delayed reaction to previous traumas

The death of a loved one

Melanie's father died a week after she discovered she was pregnant with her first child. It was not until she gave birth seven months later that she finally started to grieve.

Melanie's story

'When I found out I was pregnant I was absolutely ecstatic; becoming a mum was all I had ever really wanted. I was definitely not a career person. Then my dad died. I felt numb – too much to take in. Every time I wanted to cry about my dad I would think about the baby inside me and I knew I had to stay strong for her sake. I was terrified that if I got too upset it might trigger a miscarriage, or it might have some terrible effect on my baby, and I couldn't have taken another loss, it would have been too much to bear. I just bottled everything up. I blocked out what had happened to my dad and saw my baby as some kind of compensation for him dying. After my daughter was born I felt like a zombie – that's the only way I can describe it. I had this new person to love, but she was not my dad. Slowly I began to realise that he was never coming back. I started to feel as if I was losing my mind. I adored my daughter but I was terrified of something bad happening to her. I became totally paranoid about leaving her on her own or with anyone else, even for a second. I started doing really strange things, like trying to talk to my dad through my daughter as if he had somehow been reincarnated in her. When I told one of my friends the thoughts I was having she said she thought I was having some kind of breakdown and told me to get help. I was terrified and I didn't *know what to do – if I asked for help would they take my daughter away from me? I struggled on for another couple of months, but things just got worse and worse. I couldn't talk to my mum because I didn't want to burden her – she was trying to come to terms with her own loss. In the end I phoned my doctor and she was totally different from what I had expected. Instead of criticising me, she was really supportive and put me in touch with a bereavement counsellor. It's taken me a year even to start to come to terms with my dad's death, but I know I'm on the right track. My daughter will always be special to me because of what happened, but I am learning to relax a bit and not be so obsessive about her safety.'*

Bringing a new life into the world can act as a harsh reminder of those people we have lost, particularly if you have not had a chance to grieve properly. Do not feel guilty if you find yourself grieving for a loved one when you feel you should be rejoicing at the birth of your child. Instead, seek support from wherever you can find it and express the emotions you are feeling. The sooner you let these feelings out, the sooner you will come to terms with your loss and be able to move on with your life.

A previous miscarriage or stillbirth

If you have previously lost a child through miscarriage or stillbirth, becoming pregnant again can be extremely uplifting. However, once the new baby arrives all kinds of emotions can be evoked. What would your other child have looked like by now? How old would he/she be? If only he/she could have been here to see your new baby – their new brother or sister. Thoughts such as these are all signs that you have not fully come to terms with your previous loss. Perhaps bereavement counselling or talking through your feelings with a close friend or relative will help to heal these wounds and enable you to view the future with your new baby more positively.

A recent move

Moving to a new area seems to be a significant factor in both ante-natal and postnatal depression. At a time when a woman perhaps feels at her most vulnerable, she needs the security of the familiar. Moving house can be one of the most stressful experiences of mod-ern life and coming close to a pregnancy or birth can often tip the balance between feeling a bit emotional and feeling downright depressed. Cheryl suffered from both antenatal and postnatal depression. She writes:

'We recently moved to my partner's home town and I don't know anyone at all. So on my days off work I don't go any-where or do anything, I just clean our home and do the washing and ironing. I've had a very hard time trying to be positive about this baby. I desperately want to be positive, but every time I try something negative happens. I've always found comfort in shopping, but since we moved I can't afford to do this and I'm starting to feel quite resentful.'

Natalie discovered she was pregnant two weeks after moving to Ireland to be nearer her husband's family.

'My husband is gone 14 hours a day to work in Dublin, leaving me stuck in a farmhouse with his mother and my two sisters-in-law. I had all these dreams of starting my own busi-ness once we got over here, but now I've had to put them all on hold. I'm used to the hustle and bustle of city life and I just can't stand sitting around here all day, being lectured on how to be a good mum and all the things I'm doing wrong. I'm so home-sick I sometimes wish I was dead. It feels like my friends are a million miles away – I feel so cut off and isolated here.'

Leaving work

Gone are the days when a woman's sole purpose in life was to have children and create the perfect home. Women are now higher achievers than men in both education and the workplace. Having children is being put off until career goals are attained and then, after years of independence and spontaneity, the joys of parenthood can come as a huge shock.

Even women who look forward to a career break and want to bring up their children themselves, rather than leave them in the care of strangers, can find the drastic change to their lifestyle unbearable. Ginny delayed having her first child until she was 34, as she was working her way up the ranks of the civil service.

'My mother had me when she was just 21 and she went on to have another three children. As I got older I realised the sacrifices she had made by having us so young. She was so intelligent and yet she never pursued her ambitions. I think she felt it was too late for her but she really pushed me. It was taken for granted that I would be going to university and she always warned me never to get married before the age of 30. So it was natural for me to concentrate on my career. I got my degree and got a job in the civil service and spent 12 years working my way up the ladder. When I reached my thirties my biological clock started ticking rather loudly. Suddenly I became obsessed with anything to do with babies. My partner was overjoyed – I think he had given up hope of us ever starting a family. So I decided I would take at least five years off work to bring up my child until he was ready for school and possibly have another one. By the time I left work I was really looking forward to the break – I rather naïvely imagined it would all be walks in the park and lullabies – I hadn't prepared myself for the loneliness and frustration I would feel. All my friends were still working and I felt completely isolated stuck at home with my baby. Although I loved my baby I also began to resent him. I would spend hours wondering what they were doing at work. My mind seemed to go stale. I had nobody to talk to and nothing to challenge me. I felt a complete failure, both as a mother and career wise. My health *visitor recommended I join a mother and baby group that held coffee mornings once a week. At first I found the idea very unappealing – a load of mums sitting around comparing notes about their babies, but in the end I got so desperate for some company I decided to give it a go. I was really shy at first as my depression had caused me to lose a lot of self-confidence. After a couple of weeks I started to look forward to going. A couple of the women were from very similar backgrounds to me and we started to meet up separately, taking it in turns to go round to each others' houses with a bottle of wine. By the time my son was a year old I'd got a part time job as a Saturday receptionist and my husband looked after our son. It certainly wasn't a career move, but I just needed to get out and meet people. This way I can have the best of both worlds.'*

The social causes of postnatal depression

Returning to work

One of the major changes in our society of recent times has been the role of women in the workplace. Many women work extremely hard to establish a career and enjoy the challenges and motivation that this provides. They are then faced with a very difficult decision when they start a family – should they put their career on hold for at least five years and miss out on the stimulation that work provides, or should they return to work and experience the wrench of leaving their baby in the care of others? The issue of work seems to crop up quite regularly in cases of postnatal depression, but in various different ways. Valerie was a senior account manager in a male-dominated industry when she became pregnant with her only son.

'I knew before I had even fallen pregnant that I would be returning to work at the earliest possible opportunity. I had worked long and hard to get where I was and was proud of the fact that I had made it as a woman in what was a predominantly male environment. I worked right through my

pregnancy and as soon as my son was six weeks old I took him to a nursery and returned to work. Within a week I was feeling depressed. I found it increasingly hard to focus on work. It wasn't that I was tired – I'm one of those lucky people who can survive on four hours sleep a night – I was very anxious all the time. My job involved travelling around the country and I hated being so far away from my baby. I was terrified that something might happen to him; that he would need me and I wouldn't be able to get to him in time. People in the office seemed to treat me differently as well. I may have been being a bit paranoid, but I felt as if they were judging me, that they thought I was an uncaring mother – particularly the other female staff. As I got more depressed my work rate inevitably suffered and for the first time in my career my boss called me in to give me a warning. I realised then that I had to do something. Luckily my company were in the process of down-sizing so I decided to take advantage of the voluntary redundancy package that was on offer. I knew I wouldn't be happy without some form of work so I used my redundancy money to set up a small business based from my home. Although it can get pretty hectic at times I am happy that I have my son with me now, and on the odd occasion that I do need to go out to an appointment my husband takes time off to look after him.'

Returning to work is not always the cause of postnatal depression; in many cases it seems to be the cure, as the following examples demonstrate:

'I'm not sure if I was suffering from clinical depression, but my mind was certainly miserable and confused for about nine months after the birth of my child. I only truly felt better after I returned to work. I remember being so grateful for the chance to go out and not be "chained" to the house.'

'I was reluctant to use the word "depression" in relation to the birth of my first child, referring to it instead as "fed up", or "feeling a bit low", but in retrospect I'm sure it was postnatal depression. I never sought any help for it and fortunately I managed to overcome it by returning to work and "normality".'

Both examples highlight what a shock to the system giving up your job can be. Although bringing up a baby undoubtedly involves a lot of hard work, it also usually involves long periods of time without any sort of interaction with other adults, so loneliness can easily set in. If you feel your postnatal depression may be linked to leaving work ask yourself the following questions:

- Do you long for other, adult company?
- Do you feel as if your mind is becoming stagnant?
- Do you long for some kind of mental challenge?
- Do you feel your baby is suffering because you are so unhappy?
- Have you considered doing a part-time course, either in the evening or from home?
- Is there any type of work that you could do on a freelance basis from home?
- Do you know of a child-minder or a nursery where you could leave your child and not have any concerns for their safety or well-being?

If you answer 'Yes' to the majority of these questions then the key to a quick recovery from postnatal depression probably lies in returning to some form of work, be it full- or part-time or some type of academic or training course. Having a child could actually prove to be the perfect chance to pursue a completely different career path, also providing more opportunity to be with your baby.

The breakdown of the extended family

As with antenatal depression, the breakdown of the extended family plays a significant role in the incidence of postnatal depression. In more traditional societies, such as Japan, childbirth is still taken very seriously. Extensive preparations are made throughout the pregnancy and the woman returns to live with her own mother for the first few months after the birth. Consequently, the number and severity of cases of postnatal depression are significantly lower than in Western society.

In today's society women have higher expectations than ever placed upon them and yet are faced with ever dwindling support. The help traditionally provided by the extended family needs to be replaced by other sources, such as better postnatal care, support groups and organisations.

The isolation and despair of postnatal depression

'I became terrified that I might do something to hurt my baby; that I might lose control for a few seconds and do something terrible. I dreaded being left on my own with him – I couldn't cope any more, but I felt like there was nowhere to turn. How could I possibly admit to the thoughts I'd been having?'

'For months I struggled on refusing to admit to myself I needed help. I'd never experienced any form of depression before, not even PMT, and I thought I must be cracking up. I thought if I told anyone about the way I was feeling they'd lock me up and throw away the key.'

'When I told my friends the way I'd been feeling they looked at me as if I'd gone mad. "How can you not be happy – you've just had a baby?" they'd ask. In the end I gave up trying to explain and kept everything bottled up inside.'

These are just a few of the comments from sufferers of postnatal depression that highlight the fear and isolation they experienced. As with antenatal depression there is still a great deal of stigma attached to feeling negative about the birth of your child. Unlike antenatal depression, however, there is a support group to which sufferers can turn. The Association for Postnatal Illness is a helpline offering confidential support and advice, putting women in touch with a volunteer who has herself recovered from postnatal depression. The National Childbirth Trust, the largest and best-known childbirth and parenting charity in Europe, has also provided many sufferers of postnatal depression with invaluable support. Please see the Useful Addresses section on page 171 of this book for further information.

A study of postnatal depression carried out in 1996 showed that 90 per cent of sufferers realised that there was something wrong but fewer than 20 per cent actually reported it to a member of the medical profession.[3] As with antenatal depression, fear and embarrassment are preventing women from seeking help, and yet proper assistance, early on, is essential for a speedy recovery and return to normality.

Chapter 4
The Effects of Antenatal and Postnatal Depression Upon the Partner

Men are all too often the forgotten victims of antenatal and postnatal depression. Becoming a father can have a huge impact on a man and yet all the attention seems to be focused upon the mother. Men are expected to be more interested in changing a tyre than changing a nappy and they are certainly not expected to demonstrate any kind of emotional turmoil. Consequently, rather than risk the ridicule of their friends, fathers tend to keep their fears and concerns firmly to themselves.

The Pressures of Pregnancy and Birth Upon the Father

- Increased responsibility, often as the sole breadwinner
- Feeling left out
- Exhaustion from a combination of sleep deprivation and having to work
- Lack of support or flexibility in the workplace
- Less attention or affection from partner
- Less freedom

When these pressures are combined with their partner's unexpect-ed depression, either during or after pregnancy (or both), the father is often thrown into turmoil himself. At a time when he expected to be feeling happy and excited he finds himself going through the following emotions:

- **Fear** at partner's apparent loss of control
- **Hurt** at believing they are somehow the cause of their partner's depression
- **Rejection** at partner's loss of interest in sex or any other physical affection
- **Confusion** at partner's negativity at a time that is supposed to be joyful
- **Helplessness,** unsure of how to act or what to do for the best
- **Anger** at lack of available support

The following quotes from different fathers demonstrate each of these feelings in more detail:

Tom

'Cathy had always been so calm and laid back – it was really frightening to see her start to fall apart. She was the calming influence in our relationship, the one who kept our family going, but after the birth of our third child she just seemed to lose it. There were times when I seriously thought we were coming apart at the seams – I could see us ending in divorce and the kids ending up in care.'

Clive

'The worst part about my wife's antenatal depression is that I feel somehow it must be my fault. Surely if she was happy with me she would not be so depressed at the thought of having our child?'

Matty

'I know this sounds selfish, but I want my old girlfriend back. The one who used to be all over me. These days I'm lucky if I get a word out of her let alone a kiss or a hug.'

Neil

'We had been planning this baby for months and when my girlfriend finally became pregnant I was made up. Right from the start though she was miserable. She didn't stop crying and worrying about every little thing. I couldn't understand it – I thought she had wanted a baby as much as I did.'

Stefan

'It wasn't until I read the article on antenatal depression that I felt any sort of hope. When my wife showed it to me and explained that this was what was happening to her I finally had some kind of understanding. Until that point I didn't know if it was something I was doing wrong or wasn't doing at all that was causing her depression. I sometimes wondered if she was cracking up – I just didn't know what to think.'

Darren

'When my wife got postnatal depression after the birth of our second child I was obviously very upset at first, but after a while I have to admit that I did get a bit annoyed and resentful. Everything in all the books and magazines seems to be about supporting the woman. My wife ended up having counselling once a week, but there was nobody there for me. At times I was having to look after all four of us and hold down a full-time job. The house would be a mess when I got in from work and I'd have to do the tea and feed the kids, but nobody wanted to help me out.'

Depression in the Father

Many men find themselves feeling quite depressed after the birth of their child. Becoming a parent can be just as traumatic for the father as it can for the mother, yet there is even less support available to them. If women feel too ashamed or embarrassed to seek professional help they can still cry on the shoulders of their friends or close relatives. This is not the case for men. The only time it is socially acceptable for a man to say he is depressed is in relation to his football team losing or his horse coming last.

Steve describes the double life he was forced to lead when his wife fell victim to postnatal depression shortly after the birth of their first child:

> 'At work I was still Jack-the-lad – I work in a warehouse with 15 other blokes – there was no way I could have ever told any of them how I was really feeling. If I'd walked into the tea room and said, "I'm feeling a bit down today lads, go easy on the banter", I'd have been crucified. So I'd pretend there was nothing wrong all day then come home to find my wife sitting there in the darkness just crying. The house would be a mess and there would be nothing for my tea. I felt terrible. I knew I should be doing something to help her, but I didn't know what. Nothing I did or said seemed to help. I dreaded going home and, yes, on some nights I had a bloody good cry myself – not that I'd have ever told anyone. If truth be told I was probably more frightened than I'd ever been in my whole life.'

With no one there to support them, fathers may well find it increasingly difficult to support their partners. This leads to relationships becoming stretched to breaking point at a time when both partners need each other most.

Steps to Take if your Partner is Suffering from Antenatal or Postnatal Depression

Many former sufferers of antenatal and postnatal depression speak in glowing terms about the love and support they received from their partners. Here are just some examples:

Lisa

'I am so lucky; I must have a husband in a million to have put up with what he did. Every weekend when he was home from work I would tear into him; everything would be his fault. One time I even attacked him physically. It was as if I was taking all my frustration out on him. No matter what I did or how bad it got he just stayed patient and was always there for me.'

Jenny

'Luckily I have a very patient and caring husband who has stood by me, even though at times I didn't want him around as I wanted to wallow in self-pity. He has seen me through two very stressful pregnancies. He has put up with my foul moods, anxiety and severe panic attacks.'

Alison

'Some nights I would lie in bed crying for hours on end. Steve would ask me what was wrong and would try to cuddle me, but I would just push him away. He hadn't done anything but I couldn't bring myself to talk to him, I couldn't bear to have him touch me. With hindsight I don't know how he put up with it. I must have been a complete nightmare to live with.'

So how can you provide the support that your partner so badly needs? First, it is imperative that you receive sufficient support yourself. Unfortunately there are no helplines or support groups for the partners of sufferers of antenatal or postnatal depression, but your GP will probably be able to answer most of your concerns. Alternatively, an older friend or relative may be able to offer advice. The most important thing is that you are able to express your fears and frustrations and do not bottle them up. It is also worth using the following pointers as a guide to how to act and what sort of things to do or say to your partner. Remember, the more supportive you are the more likely she is to make a speedy recovery.

- **Allow her to express her feelings** even if they make no sense to you or seem completely illogical. Remember that she is suffering from depression and will be viewing things in a completely different way from normal.

- **Remain calm and patient** even if you are faced with extreme provocation. Your partner will be feeling afraid and frustrated and lashing out at you may be her only way of expressing herself.

- **Do not take physical rejection personally.** When your partner is feeling drained and depressed physical affection or sex is often the last thing on her mind. This is not a sign that she no longer loves you, it is a symptom of her illness and should be treated as such.

- **Go out together without the children.** As soon as possible after the birth of your baby take your partner out on her own. Even if it is just for a couple of hours, for a meal or a drink, it will remind her of how things used to be and allow you some time together to talk.

- **Communicate.** Rather than avoiding one another and living in silence talk about your feelings. Tell her how you are feeling, and about any insecurities you may have. Try to encourage her to open up to you.

- **Offer sympathy and support** even if you are feeling resentful or under pressure yourself. Allow her to feel unconditional love and this will make her feel stronger.

- **Allow your partner some regular time for herself.** You could offer to look after the baby every Saturday morning, giving her time to see a friend, do some shopping or have her hair done. This will give her something to look forward to every week.

- **Acknowledge any effort she makes,** however small. For instance, if you notice the house looks tidier or she has made more of an effort with the tea, be sure to comment positively.

- **Praise her parenting skills.** Comment on what a good mother she will make/makes. Back this up with examples.

- **Seek help for yourself.** Remember this is not just about the mother; as a father you have needs and feelings too. Seek help from wherever you can find it.

The key thing for both parents to remember in all of this is that you are partners. It is all too easy to fall into the trap of blaming and resenting each other, but that will get you nowhere. By sticking together you will help each other through this difficult period in your lives and face the future a stronger, more committed partnership.

Chapter 5
The Effects of Antenatal and Postnatal Depression Upon the Baby

Most sufferers of antenatal and postnatal depression worry about the effects their illness may be having on their baby. *'I've been so anxious and moody all pregnancy, I just know I'm going to give birth to a nervous wreck'*, appears to be a common concern for sufferers of antenatal depression. Sufferers of postnatal depression tend to worry about the long-term damage that may have been caused by their inability to bond with their child or show any kind of enthusiasm in the first few months of their development.

The Effects of Antenatal Depression Upon the Unborn Child

Studies of antenatal depression and its effects upon the foetus have only started in the last ten years and much more research is needed. However, the studies that have been carried out have found that depression and anxiety in the pregnant woman can have the following effects upon the unborn child:

- The stress hormone cortisol may be transmitted from the mother to the baby via the placenta in sufficient amounts to affect the foetus.
- Maternal anxiety in the third trimester has been linked to

impaired blood flow in the uterine arteries; this in turn has been linked to growth restriction in the baby.

• There is an increased likelihood of premature birth and low birth weight, with all the health implications that they involve.

Jessica describes what she believes to be the outcome of her antenatal depression:

> 'Three years ago, whilst expecting my first baby, and when seven months pregnant, I became very depressed and scared. Eventually I asked my doctor for some counselling, but before this was arranged I gave birth (two weeks early). I am convinced the depression and high state of anxiety I was in brought the birth forward.'

Although there is a desperate need for more research to be carried out in this area, most existing studies have shown a link between antenatal depression and babies being born earlier and smaller for their gestational age. A review of several recent studies, carried out at Queen Charlotte's Hospital in London, concludes that:

> 'We suggest two possible mechanisms by which maternal anxiety or stress may be communicated to and affect the foetus; (i) direct transport of cortisol across the placenta, and (ii) impaired blood flow through the uterine arteries. We do not yet know at which stages of pregnancy these are likely to have the greatest effects, nor the extent to which they explain the epidemiological and animal studies linking maternal stress/anxiety with adverse outcome such as smaller and lower gestational age babies, and children with later behavioural problems. Appropriate interventions to reduce antenatal maternal stress or anxiety may well have a long term beneficial effect on the child.'[1]

Sufferers of antenatal depression have a right to know the results of these studies and equally they have a right to expect a far better support network than currently exists. If you are suffering from antenatal depression it is vitally important that you do not allow these facts to become another cause of anxiety or concern; instead let them encourage you to seek help. The medical profession is far more aware of the problem these days and most GPs or midwives will be only too glad to offer advice and support.

Although it has also been suggested that sufferers of antenatal depression give birth to cranky, irritable babies, this is by no means a foregone conclusion. Many women have spoken of their joy and relief when, despite feeling anxious and stressed throughout their pregnancy, they finally gave birth to a cheerful, contented baby.

Rosie

'I have to admit on more than one occasion I wondered what the hell I was going to give birth to. I had been so miserable and moody for most of my pregnancy that I was sure it would have had an affect upon my baby's personality. I couldn't have been more wrong. Liam was a delightful baby, an excellent sleeper and such a happy little chap. I couldn't have wished for a better child.'

The Effects of Postnatal Depression Upon the Baby

Eve

'Although I got over my postnatal depression years ago I am still haunted by the fear that it will have had some lasting effect on my daughter. I remember not being able to do anything with her when we first came home from the hospital. I would just sit and stare at her when she cried; I really had no maternal urges at all. For the nine months I was depressed I wandered around in a daze. I didn't have any other feelings apart from an overwhelming sense of gloom. I had been

*expecting to have all of this unconditional love for her imme-
diately, but to be completely honest it wasn't until Ella was
about a year old that I started feeling any kind of love towards
her at all. She is five years old now and we get on very well,
but sometimes I wonder if she can remember what a terrible
mother I was for that first year. Would we have been closer if
I hadn't got depressed? I'll never know, but it will always
worry me.'*

Postnatal depression has been likened to falling into a deep well
of despair. As the sufferer sinks further and further down they find
it increasingly hard to reach out to others on the outside, including
their own baby. The feelings Eve has described are typical of most
sufferers. The inability to bond and the lack of any kind of positive
interaction with their babies leave mothers feeling guilty about any
long-term damage they may be causing. Many studies have been
carried out on the effects, both short- and long-term, of postnatal
depression upon the baby, with the following findings.

Short-term effects

- **Withdrawal.** Some babies will become withdrawn and will stop
  expecting or demanding attention from their mothers.

- **Hyperactivity.** Other babies will go to the opposite extreme, trying harder and harder to get attention, crying incessantly and
  displaying anger at being neglected.

Long-term effects

- **Problematic relationship.** Long after the postnatal depression
  has gone its legacy can live on in a difficult and insecure relationship between the mother and child.

- **Behaviour.** There is an increased risk of children going on to
  suffer from behavioural problems later in life.

- **Lower IQ.** The latest study on the long-term effects of postnatal depression upon the child has highlighted a worrying link with lower IQ. This link is strongest in cases where the mother suffered from depression in the first three months after the birth and appears to affect boys far more than girls. The sons of sufferers of postnatal depression studied had an average IQ score of 86 – considerably lower than the average of 103 scored by the sons of non-depressed mothers. There was only a four point difference between the groups of girls studied, with IQ scores of 94 and 98.[2]

It is important that women suffering from postnatal depression do not become too alarmed by these findings. Many other factors need to be taken into consideration. The sooner the woman's depression is diagnosed and treated, the better the chances of no long-term side-effects occurring. A lot is also dependent on the child's surroundings, the role that other members of the family play and the baby's own character. As with antenatal depression these findings should not be used as another reason to feel guilt or despair, but rather as an incentive to seek help and support.

Chapter 6
Seeking Medical Help

Breaking the Cycle of Despair

Once you fall victim to depression you find yourself trapped in a cycle of despair that can be extremely hard to break out of. This may be the reason that some sufferers of antenatal depression go on to experience postnatal depression and why cases of postnatal depression usually last long after the sleepless nights and initial chaos have died down. As a sufferer of depression you are likely to experience some or all of the following things:

- Self-loathing and a general lack of self-worth
- Dislike of others in general
- Constantly seeing the negative side of events and thinking negative thoughts
- Inability to experience any emotions other than a dull numbness and despondency
- General feeling of lethargy, lack of energy or enthusiasm for anything
- Problems sleeping, either inability to sleep or difficulties waking up
- Problems with eating, either by binging on unhealthy food or losing appetite completely
- Turning to stimulants such as tobacco, caffeine, alcohol or other drugs
- Isolating yourself from the outside world and refusing to seek help.

All these traits end up becoming self-fulfilling prophecies and in doing so perpetuate the cycle of despair. For example:

You dislike yourself as a person
↓
You avoid other people
↓
You are seen as hostile
↓
Others reject or ignore you
↓
You feel that this is what you deserve
↓
You dislike yourself

Before long your whole life is revolving around your depression. So how can you break free of this cycle and find things to smile about once more? In this section of the book we will look at the different ways in which sufferers of antenatal or postnatal depression can help themselves, first by seeking medical help.

Overcoming the Fear of Seeking Professional Help

Many women are too afraid to tell their doctor or midwife about their depression. Rather than seeking help at the earliest possible opportunity they wait until it becomes too much to bear, or struggle on without any help at all. A review of postnatal depression carried out in 1997 estimated that only 20 per cent of sufferers receive any kind of mental health treatment.[1] The reasons for women's reluctance to come forward can be broken down into the following three areas:

- Shame or embarrassment at having negative feelings towards pregnancy and birth
- Fear that they will be deemed unfit to be a mother
- General fear or suspicion of authority.

Nikki explains her refusal to seek help for antenatal depression:

'The only thing I could find written on the subject of ante-natal depression was a brief mention in a book that said the main cause was the mother not wanting her baby. I knew this was not the reason for my feeling so low – I desperately want-ed my baby, but I thought that if I did go and see my doctor he would think that I didn't. I thought my child might have ended up on an "at risk" register.'

The health service is starting to address this problem by providing more intensive antenatal and postnatal check-ups, focusing on how the mother is coping mentally as well as physically. Questionnaires are being introduced at the routine postnatal six-week check, asking the mother to describe any doubts, fears and anxieties she may be having. It is important that you answer these questions honestly in order that you can receive the help you need. You will not be condemned as an unfit mother, nor will your child be taken away from you. This chapter looks in detail at the various sources of support and advice on offer from the health service.

Antidepressants

Although most doctors are reluctant to offer antidepressants during pregnancy (due to the risk of damage to the foetus) they are quite commonly used in the treatment of postnatal depression. Many women are wary of being prescribed medication for fear of becoming addicted, but they are worrying unnecessarily. Unlike tranquillisers, antidepressants are non-addictive drugs which work by correcting the chemical imbalances in the brain caused by depression. They do not target the cause of the depression, but rather the symptoms. However, this can be just enough to allow you to break out of the cycle of despair and get your life back on track again, as Marion found:

'When I saw my doctor about my postnatal depression she immediately prescribed me Prozac. I was nervous at first. I

had never suffered from depression before and I didn't know the first thing about antidepressants. I was scared that there could be horrific side-effects or that I might end up addicted for life, but once my doctor explained the facts I decided to give it a go. It was another four weeks before I noticed any real improvement, but suddenly I started to feel a sense of well-being and serenity that I hadn't felt for a long, long time. I was on Prozac for three months altogether and I don't regret it for a moment. It allowed me to see things in a positive light again and gave me hope at a time when I needed it most.'

There are various antidepressants that may be prescribed to sufferers of postnatal depression. Please see below for a brief description of how they work and any potential side-effects. It is

Name	How they work	Potential side-effects
Trycyclic (TCAs)	Stop the chemicals serotonin and noradrenaline (the 'feel good' chemicals) from being reabsorbed into the brain cells, leaving more to circulate and improve mood	Drowsiness, confusion, constipation, tingling sensation, blurred vision
Monoamine Oxidase Inhibitors (MAOIs)	Prevent the breakdown of the 'feel good' chemicals	Various dietary restrictions with older versions
Selective Serotonin Re-uptake Inhibitors (SSRIs)	Such as Prozac; increase the levels of serotonin in the brain	Fewer side-effects, but can reduce sex drive and cause headaches and nausea
Lithium	A mood stabiliser for severe manic depression	Can be toxic if levels are too high; has to be closely monitored

important to remember that everyone's body chemistry is different and we respond to the different antidepressants accordingly. If you experience unpleasant side-effects to a particular drug your GP will prescribe a more suitable alternative.

Counselling

Counselling is the preferred first step in most GPs' treatment of antenatal depression – it is also used for mild cases of postnatal depression. The sufferer is referred to a counsellor, with whom she has to attend regular meetings. These meetings give the victim of antenatal or postnatal depression an ideal opportunity to express themselves. It is often easier to be totally honest with a complete stranger than it is to a close friend or partner. The counsellor will listen sympathetically and then offer advice catered specifically to the woman's needs. Counselling tends to focus on the current situation and will not usually look into your past history. It is usually a short-term treatment designed to get you through short-term feelings of depression.

Psychotherapy

If your GP believes that your depression may actually be linked to your own behaviour, your low self-worth or a more deep-rooted problem from your past, you will probably be referred to a psychotherapist rather than a counsellor. The most effective form of therapy for sufferers of antenatal and postnatal depression is cognitive behavioural therapy.

The key element to cognitive behavioural therapy is getting the mother to examine and take control of her own behaviour. Women are taught to become aware of every time they think or act in a negative way and to counter it with a more positive thought or action. Rather than simply providing a listening ear or a shoulder to cry on, the therapist will play a more active role than the counsellor, intervening when the mother is being negative, highlighting any self-criticism and demonstrating how past events may be playing a role in the current depression. Linda received cognitive behavioural therapy when her antenatal depression became too much to bear:

'My therapist taught me how to feel proud of myself again. I had been plagued by self-doubt and insecurity throughout my pregnancy and the simplest thing had become a major ordeal. If I had a pile of ironing to do I would just sit and stare at it – using it as another reason to feel useless and no good. But my therapist taught me to praise myself for any achievement I made, however small. If I managed to get just one shirt ironed I had to focus on that achievement rather than the pile that remained unironed.'

Exercises in Cognitive Behavioural Therapy

There are many different exercises in cognitive behavioural therapy designed to break the cycle of negativity in which sufferers of depression find themselves. Here are just some examples.

Exercise one

Keep a record of negative thoughts and actions

Keep a daily record of your negative thought processes. It is important that you do this every day so that you can monitor any improvements. Divide each day into the following categories:

- **Situation.** Describe an event that has occurred to make you feel depressed. *For example: your inability to stop your baby crying.*

- **Feelings aroused.** List the emotions this situation caused you to feel. *For example: 'anger, frustration, despair'.*

- **Action.** Write down what action you then took. *For example: 'I started to cry', or 'I left the room.'*

- **Beliefs.** What did this situation lead you to believe about yourself. *For example: 'I'm a terrible mother', or 'I can't do anything right.'*

- **Justify your beliefs.** Think rationally about yourself as a person and try to find evidence to support your beliefs. *For example: Is it really true that you are a terrible mother? Don't all babies cry? Not everything you do is a mistake.*

- **Real reason for negativity.** Write down what you now perceive to be the real reason for your negative thoughts. *For example:'over-tiredness', or 'jumping to the wrong conclusion'.*

When you initially record the feelings that were aroused rate them from 0–10 in intensity, with 10 being the strongest. After you have completed the real reason for your negativity go back to the feelings aroused: how would you rate those feelings now? By working through a negative situation in this way you are enabling yourself to reduce your feelings of frustration or despair. When attempting to justify your beliefs it is important to examine the situation thoroughly. In the example used of the baby who would not stop crying the mother should ask herself the following questions:

- Do other babies cry?
- Do other mothers always manage to silence a crying baby instantly?
- Would your friends and relatives think you were a bad mother simply because your baby was crying?
- What other reasons could there be for your baby to cry?
- Is your baby permanently crying?
- In the grand scheme of events, is your baby crying briefly really all that terrible?
- Is there any concrete evidence to back this up?

Exercise two

Write a life chart

Starting from your earliest recollections, write a life chart concentrating on all the negative or disruptive things that have happened to you, such as your parents divorcing, the death of a loved one or the discovery of a partner's infidelity. Then write a detailed account of how each event affected you and how you coped at the time. Did you express these feelings at the time of the event or are they still bottled up? Becoming a mother is an emotionally-charged event, and many past traumas may well be revisited. If you do identify one or more problems from your past that were never properly resolved this may well be at the root of your antenatal or post-natal depression. By working through these events with a therapist you will finally relieve yourself of the burdens from your past and be able to face a brighter future.

Exercise three

Self portraits

Write a self portrait. What kind of person do you perceive yourself to be? What are your strengths? What are your weaknesses? The depressed person will usually list far more weaknesses than strengths and a self portrait is likely to be highly self critical. Now re-write the portrait of yourself as though it were by a close friend or relative. How do they perceive you? Would they identify the same weaknesses or would they see far more strengths? In this way you are learning to view yourself from an outside perspective rather than constantly looking inwards.

Exercise four

Keep a diary

Keep a diary close at hand and each time you are feeling particularly depressed write down exactly how you are feeling. At the end

of each day go over what you have written and counter each negative statement with something positive. For instance, if at lunch
time you had written, '*This house is a tip, I'm never going to find
the time to hoover*', in the evening you could counter this with,
'*But I did manage to cook the tea and make sure the baby was fed.*'
Give each day a mark out of 10 to reflect your general mood, with
0 being the most depressed and 10 being the happiest. Over the
weeks a gradual improvement in these marks will provide you with
encouragement that you are conquering your depression.

Exercise five

'Prove it !'

Get into the habit of challenging every negative thought that you
have. This becomes easier with practice, and after a while you will
become very aware of it happening. Each time ask yourself to 'prove
it'. Examples of the kinds of negative thoughts common to sufferers
of antenatal and postnatal depression are as follows:

- I'll never make a good mother
- I'm letting my partner down
- I'm a complete failure
- My life is over now I'm a mother
- I'll never lose this weight
- My partner doesn't love me or find me attractive any more
- I'll never bond with my baby
- I know my baby will be born physically or mentally handi-
  capped
- I know there will be complications with the birth
- I'm of no value to anyone now that I no longer work
- My baby will never love me if I return to work after the birth

Each time you find yourself thinking one of these thoughts ask
yourself to prove it. Write down the thought on a piece of
paper and list all the things you can think of to back it up. For
example:

- My baby will no longer love me if I return to work after the birth.
  Proof: *'I read somewhere that the children of working mums become more attached to their child-minder and resent their mothers neglecting them.'*

Is this really proof? Surely you will not be spending all your time at work? Why will a child not bond with a happy, loving mother with whom he spends evenings, weekends and holidays?

- My partner doesn't love me or find me attractive any more.
  Proof: *'He seems distant and he never wants to have sex any more.'*

Again, question your proof. How have you been acting towards him? Perhaps he is too afraid to approach you for fear of upsetting you even further. Have you asked him why he no longer wants to have sex? A lot of men are scared that sex during pregnancy may damage the unborn child, or scared of being rejected by a partner suffering from postnatal depression, assuming that sex would be the last thing on her mind.

Exercise six

Stopping the domino effect of depression

As we have previously seen, depression can become a cycle of negative thoughts and it can also create a domino effect. One small negative thought can quickly trigger off larger ones, similar to the effect of one domino causing the whole line to collapse. For example, a simple mistake such as burning some toast can easily lead to the far more serious feeling that you are unfit to be a mother, as the following example demonstrates:

- You burn a slice of toast
  (the non-depressed person simply throws it in the bin and makes another)
- The depressed person thinks, 'I'm a terrible cook'
  (the non-depressed person relaxes with her second piece of toast)

- The depressed person begins to sob as she thinks, 'If I can't even make a piece of toast how can I ever be a good mother?' (the non-depressed person finishes her toast and gets on with her day)
- The depressed person spends the next few hours crying over what a failure she is as a person.

This example demonstrates quite clearly the difference in thought processes between the depressed and the non-depressed, and how much time is wasted on simply feeling depressed. The point of this exercise is to learn gradually to stop the domino effect. Every time something minor goes wrong react accordingly. If you burn the toast, simply throw it in the bin and make another and mentally stop yourself from thinking anything more negative than, 'Oh bother!' (or another, more suitable curse).

Exercise seven

Develop a 'feel good' list
Compile a list of all those things that make you feel good. If you are feeling depressed you may find this a little difficult so here are some ideas to help you:

- Talking to a particular friend
- Going for a walk
- Going for a jog
- Dancing
- Listening to music
- Watching a good comedy
- A particular food
- Some form of beauty treatment, such as a haircut or facial
- Taking a long relaxing bath
- Writing
- Reading
- Drawing
- Poetry

When you are pregnant, and particularly after you have given birth, your whole life centres around caring for another person/other people. It is important that you do not ignore your own needs, so every day try to make use of your 'feel good' list to meet these needs:

First, every time you feel negative about something try to counter it by doing one of the things on your list.

Second, make a point of singling out one thing from your list to do each day. This will automatically give you something to look forward to, even if it is as simple as hiring yourself a good video.

Other Exercises in Self-help

There are many other exercises in self-help that you can try out at home. Here are just some, tailored specifically to the needs of the sufferer of antenatal and postnatal depression.

The trauma of leaving work

Leaving work or the prospect of leaving work can lead to the following negative feelings:

- Loss of self confidence and sense of identity
- Isolation at having no adult company
- Lack of mental stimulation or challenges

Try the following exercises to turn the negative experience of leaving work into something more positive.

Exercise eight

Visualise your ideal future

You will not be stuck at home forever. Now is an ideal time to take stock of your life and make plans for your own future. Pick a peaceful moment (this may take some time!) and relax with your eyes closed. Count slowly from 10 backwards in order to clear your mind of thoughts of nappy wipes and sterilising solution and when you begin to feel calmer visualise yourself living your ideal life. Picture your surroundings, and your own appearance. Where will you be working? Who will you be with? Allow your imagination to run free. It is important to stay vaguely in touch with reality – if your husband looks like Jack Duckworth there is little point visualising him as Jack Nicholson (unless divorce figures in your future plans!). Think of the type of lifestyle you always dreamed of leading. Then take a piece of paper and a pen and write down a five-year plan of how you might achieve this lifestyle. You might view this exercise as little more than indulging in a pipe dream, but the following example demonstrates how effectively it can work.

Once upon a time a woman found herself the victim of postnatal depression. She would spend hours on end in her North London flat feeling that her life had ground to a standstill. She no longer had a career or financial independence, she missed her friends, and her husband was more interested in supporting his football team than his depressed wife. One day when reality had become too much to bear she sat down and visualised her ideal life. Being a writer was something she had always longed to do so she pictured herself sitting at her keyboard, working on her latest novel while her son played happily in the garden of her home in the country. She then pictured her husband coming home and announcing that he hated football and would never again mention Wolverhampton Wanderers.

The woman then set about writing her five-year plan. This involved enrolling on a correspondence course in freelance journalism, studying from home while her baby slept. Once she had completed her course she began to send her work out to various editors. Did the plan work and her visualisation become a reality? Well she started to have articles and short stories published within weeks of finishing her course. Then she and her husband decided to sell up and move to a village in the country and you are currently reading her first book. Her husband still supports Wolves, but then you can't have it all, can you?

Exercise nine

How to develop your five-year plan

Once you have a clear idea in your head of your visualised life, you need to create a realistic and achievable five-year plan.

1. Take five sheets of paper, entitling them 'Year One', 'Year Two', 'Year Three', 'Year Four' and 'Year Five'.
2. On another, blank sheet of paper, write a brief description of your ideal life at the bottom and then, starting from the top, mark out a plan to get you to your goal. If you have more than one goal you may like to divide the page into three sections. For example, if your visualisation involved a career change, a different environment and a new image, your plan might look something like this:

Career
Enrol on and complete correspondence course in public relations > Work out study timetable around the baby > Complete course > Compile list of potential customers > Approach these companies with publicity ideas > Obtain first account > **Become freelance public relations consultant**

Home life
Talk to husband > Discuss possible places to move to > Look into property prices > Redecorate current home in preparation for sale > Start viewing houses in desired area > Make appointment with building society > Arrange finances > Put property on the market and make an offer on new house > **Move house**

Appearance
Decide upon new hairstyle > fix up hair appointment > Devise exercise plan to get old figure back > Work out exercise timetable around the baby > Buy healthier foods > Cut back on junk food > Buy new clothes > **Back in shape and confident about appearance**

---

3. Looking at the different areas of your life you want to change, take the page entitled 'Year One' and decide how much you could realistically achieve within the first year. For example:

Year One
Career
Enrol on and complete public relations course
Home life
Talk to husband > Discuss possible places to move to > Look into property prices
Appearance
Decide upon new hairstyle > fix up hair appointment > Devise exercise plan to get old figure back > Work out exercise timetable around the baby > Buy healthier foods > Cut back on junk food > Buy new clothes > **Back in shape and confident about appearance**

Continue this process for all five years if you have to, until you have a detailed plan of how you can achieve each goal. The most important thing to remember is to set yourself completely realistic targets. If you aim to do too much in the first year you will only be adding to the stress and pressure you are under. Also bear in mind that the first year with a new baby is undoubtedly the most tiring so try to make Year One's targets particularly easy to achieve. This is an important exercise because it will help you to start looking to the future with hope rather than stagnating in your present despair. Each time you feel yourself sinking down into the gloom take a few minutes by yourself, visualising your ideal life and reminding yourself that you are taking steps to achieve that life. In this way you are also regaining control over your life (usually the first victim of depression).

Exercise ten

Making the most of being at home

As the long-term unemployed will confirm, there is often nothing more soul-destroying than being stuck at home. With little reason to leave the house, you stay inside; with little reason to make an effort over your appearance or even get dressed you stay in your dressing gown. Before long you have sprouted roots in the settee and have become a slave to the daytime TV schedules. The only kind of challenge in your life is trying to get a bottle made up and a nappy changed in the commercial break during 'Jerry Springer'. After a couple of months, when your husband comes home from work and asks where his tea is, without even thinking you start waving your head from side to side, pointing in a strange manner and telling him, *'Don't even go there!'* You start looking to talk-show guests to provide the excitement in your life as you feed off the endless stream of, *'Guess what? I married my sister!'* or even *'Guess what? I married my horse!'*.

Although this can prove an entertaining and relaxing break from the office intrigue of *'Guess what? The photocopier's broken down!'*, you should not allow yourself to let this way of life continue for too long. We all need stimulation and, believe it or not, the home can actually provide a more stimulating and interesting environment than the workplace.

- **Creative therapy.** Creativity is an excellent tool, frequently used in the treatment of depression. Take the opportunity to explore your creative talents whether they be poetry, writing, drawing, music, glass painting, flower arranging or photography. You do not need to enrol on a course – libraries are full of books to help get you started. Creativity enables you to express emotions, all too often pent up by depression.

- **Broaden your mind.** Aim to learn something new every day. Read biographies of people you admire; read about subjects that have always interested you but you know little about. Again make full use of your local library – it's free, and reading is one of the few things you can do quite easily whilst breast-feeding.

- **Get out and about.** Plan different places to go. Take your baby with you to meet friends for lunch. Get to know your local parks. Take a bus somewhere new. Start off locally and, as your confidence grows, broaden your horizons. Museums, the zoo, a walk by a local canal or river, feeding the ducks – aim to do all the things you were unable to do when stuck in the workplace.

The purpose of these exercises is to look at life outside yourself. Depression is an extremely inward-looking illness. By making the most of being at home, to increase your knowledge and broaden your horizons, you are gradually shifting the emphasis away from yourself and your depression and learning to focus on the bigger picture once again.

Psychiatric Help

In cases of severe depression and postpartum psychosis the woman is referred to a psychiatrist for more intense, closely monitored treatment. Treatment is usually a combination of medication and psychotherapy, and some form of hospital attendance will also be required. This will either be as a day patient or, in more severe cases, a stay in hospital in a specialist mother-and-baby unit in order to avoid the trauma of separation. Because treatment can be so closely monitored in hospital it is usually highly effective. However, in the minority of cases that do not respond to treatment, electro-convulsive therapy may be recommended. This involves applying an electric charge to the brain. It is a controversial form of treatment, sometimes causing short-term memory loss, but in cases where medication and therapy have failed it has a high success rate in terms of instantly removing feelings of depression.

Chapter 7
Diet

When we feel depressed it is all too easy to seek comfort in the things that are bad for us. There are very few people who, on feeling a bit down, have a munch on a carrot and run around the block for a quick boost. When we become stressed or anxious we are far more likely to turn to cigarettes, alcohol and junk food. However, any comfort gained is usually quickly replaced by guilt at our over-indulgence and lack of self-control. This is made even worse for expectant or new mothers as they have the additional worry of possible ill-effects upon their baby. It is easy to see how drinking, smoking or unhealthy eating can play a role in both antenatal and postnatal depression – creating negative feelings and poor physical health. Although a healthy diet alone cannot provide a cure for this kind of depression, it certainly plays an important part in its treatment for the following three reasons:

- **Breaking the cycle of despair.** When you are depressed it is reflected in your diet in one of two ways – either by comfort eating or not bothering to eat at all. Both of these help to reinforce feelings of depression: comfort eating makes you feel guilty and full of self loathing, and going without food starves the body of energy making you feel dull and listless. By beginning to eat more healthily, it is possible to break free of this cycle, replacing negative feelings with a sense of self-respect and achievement.

- **Replacing lost nutrients.** During pregnancy and for the first few months after the birth the mother is likely to experience deficiencies in various nutrients such as iron, zinc and the B vitamins. These deficiencies are increasingly being linked to feelings of depression and can only be rectified by a well-balanced diet.

- **A source of energy.** Energy can be at an all-time low throughout pregnancy and immediately after the birth and this is particularly true for the sufferer of depression. A nutritious, well-balanced diet will provide the mother with more energy and go some way towards removing the feelings of lethargy often experienced.

This section looks at the particular dietary requirements of the sufferer of antenatal and postnatal depression with recipes and meal plans designed to be as realistic as possible. There is little point in setting yourself unachievable dietary targets, only to feel even more down when you fail to meet them. The reality of antenatal depression is that there are times when smoking a cigarette feels like the only thing that will keep you sane. Similarly, with only a few precious minutes available every day, the sufferer of postnatal depression is far more likely to grab a chocolate bar than labour over a lentil casserole. It is vital that you do not allow diet to become another reason to feel bad about yourself. As long as you meet your dietary requirements there is no need to feel guilty for the occasional lapse. By taking a well-balanced approach to food you can also have your chocolate cake and eat it.

Diet and Antenatal Depression

Pregnancy can often be the perfect excuse for poor eating habits; after years of being a slave to the scales many women see it as the ideal chance to hit the cream cakes with a vengeance. With the excuses that you are going to get fat anyway and you are having to eat for two, it can be all too easy to pile on unnecessary kilos. If you are suffering from antenatal depression, eating can become a welcome relief from your anxieties – after all, you're not allowed to drink or smoke any more. However, it isn't long before you start to worry about what harm your endless diet of chips and chocolate might be having on your baby. Sufferers of morning sickness experience similar anxieties. In many cases a healthy, well-balanced diet is impossible to keep down and once again dietary problems become a cause for concern and even depression.

Nutritional Deficiencies Caused by Pregnancy

During pregnancy the woman's need for folic acid, calcium, magnesium, zinc, iron, and vitamins C and B complex increases by 30–100 per cent. Unless your diet meets these increased needs your body's stores will become depleted and you will suffer certain physical side effects.

Iron deficiency

Anaemia, the deficiency of iron, is known to cause feelings of exhaustion and depression. Routine antenatal blood tests will detect anaemia and a high-dosage iron supplement will be prescribed. However, iron tablets have been known to cause constipation and to interfere with the body's uptake of another vital mineral, zinc. So if you can, eat plenty of iron-rich foods together with food or drinks rich in vitamin C (to increase the body's absorption of iron).

Foods rich in iron

Red meat (avoid liver, as high doses of vitamin A have been linked to birth defects)
Kidneys
Spinach, watercress and other dark green vegetables
Potato skins
Dried fruit, particularly apricots, prunes and raisins
Bananas

Molasses
Haricot beans
Cream
Cottage cheese
Egg yolks
Cocoa

Foods rich in vitamin C

Citrus fruits or juice
Kiwi fruit
Blackcurrants
Red, yellow and green vegetables
Potatoes

Zinc deficiency

Various studies have linked a deficiency in zinc to premenstrual tension, postnatal depression and problems during the menopause, so again it would make sense to include as many zinc-rich foods as possible in your diet. Lack of zinc in the diet has also been linked to morning sickness, another cause of antenatal depression.

Foods rich in zinc

Whole-wheat, wheatbran, wheatgerm, rye, oats
Shellfish
Sesame seeds
Brazil nuts
Garlic
Ginger
Leafy vegetables, watercress, onions

B complex vitamin deficiency

A deficiency of the B complex vitamins has been shown to cause feelings of anxiety and depression. As there are increased demands for this vitamin group during pregnancy it is quite easy for a deficiency to occur. Once again this increased need must be satisfied by the diet or by a B complex vitamin supplement during pregnancy.

Foods rich in B vitamins

Whole grains, wheatgerm, wheatbran, cornflour

Sunflower and sesame seeds

Brewers Yeast, Marmite spread

Kidneys

Chicken and turkey (dark meat)

Oily fish, salmon

Mushrooms, potatoes (particularly skin), green vegetables, soya beans, sweet corn

Bananas

Raisins

Cheese, eggs, milk

Foods rich in folic acid

Raw leafy vegetables, Brussels sprouts, avocado pears, broccoli

Oranges, bananas

Breakfast cereals

Walnuts

Marmite spread

Foods rich in calcium

Milk, yoghurts, fromage frais, cheese, cheese spread
Sardines
Sunflower seeds
Green vegetables

As you can see from the lists of food groups, many foods are rich in more than one vital nutrient. For example, by simply swapping from white to wholemeal bread you will instantly have a regular source of zinc, B complex vitamins and magnesium. Spread some Marmite on it and you will also be adding iron and folic acid. Wash it down with a glass of orange juice and you will be ensuring that your body absorbs all the goodness.

Morning Sickness

As previously discussed, chronic morning sickness can be a huge contributory factor to antenatal depression, and can also inevitably lead to various nutritional deficiencies. Many previously healthy women become reduced to a diet of junk food and fizzy drinks, unable to keep anything else down. Foods that they previously loved can suddenly become abhorrent and vice versa. Stephanie describes the effect her chronic sickness had upon her diet and her emotions:

'It was as if all of my tastes had been reversed overnight. I couldn't bear the smell of coffee – I would have to cross the road rather than walk past a café – and yet I had previously drunk gallons of the stuff. My diet had always been very Mediterranean – I loved pasta and vegetables, but similarly, once I became pregnant, just the smell of them would send me running for the bathroom. For the first few weeks all I could eat were plain digestive biscuits and crackers. I actually started losing weight rather than putting any on. By the time I was

*three months pregnant it had improved slightly – I could eat a
wider range of foods but it was all rubbish. I constantly craved
greasy, salty chips and still couldn't bear the thought of any
other kind of vegetable or salad. Although I had completely
gone off chocolate I would get through bags and bags of
liquorice allsorts and jelly babies. This all had a terrible effect
on my mental state. I wasn't worried so much about the effect
it was having on me – I was relieved just to be able to keep
food down – but I was much more concerned for the health of
my baby. I had read somewhere about how the foetus needs
different nutrients to develop mentally as well as physically,
and I couldn't see how my diet of chips and sweets could be
providing my baby with all that he needed. I would have nightmares about giving birth to a deformed baby – one night I even
dreamt I gave birth to a giant jelly baby! It sounds funny now,
but at the time it was all I could think about. I wanted so badly
to give my child the best possible start in life and yet I felt like
I had no choice – it was either eat rubbish or starve.'*

Stephanie's concerns are typical of many expectant mothers and
highlight how easy it is for diet to become a major cause of anxiety during pregnancy. The good news is that in the vast majority of
cases the foetus will receive all the nutrients it requires from the
mother's body. As the pregnancy progresses the mother's stores of
these nutrients will become depleted, but it is the mother who will
suffer the deficiency and not the baby.

Dietary steps to alleviate morning sickness

Try the following dietary steps in order to minimise nausea and
vomiting and the accompanying feelings of despair.

Snacks

Light snacks are usually all the sufferer of morning sickness can
stomach, but if you make these as healthy as possible they can be
just as good a source of nutrients as three main meals. Try to use

some of the following to snack on throughout the day and to keep feelings of nausea at bay. Don't worry if you also satisfy your craving for sticky buns or crisps – as long as you manage to eat some healthy food it is better than none at all.

- Dry wholemeal toast
- Wholewheat crackers and biscuits
- Wholemeal bread sandwiches
- Porridge flavoured with lemon juice or ginger marmalade
- Muesli bars (particularly those containing bran, apricot, apple, coconut)
- Nuts (peanuts should be avoided because of a potential nut allergy in the baby)
- Dried fruit, especially apricots, raisins, prunes
- Green, sharp-flavoured apples such as Granny Smiths
- Juicy, soft fruits such as peaches
- Grapes
- Any raw vegetables
- Natural, organic yoghurt, sweetened with honey or fruit purée
- Lemon sorbet
- Ginger biscuits or ginger marmalade on toast
- Sugar-free peppermints or mint-flavoured chewing gum

Drinks

Although you may crave gallons of tea, coffee and cola these all contain large amounts of caffeine, which severely reduces your body's uptake of the essential minerals iron and zinc. Try drinking the caffeine-free alternatives, or if you must have a regular 'cuppa' make sure it is between meals rather than with them. The following drinks can bring a welcome relief to feelings of nausea and add valuable nutrients to your diet:

- Lemon, ginger or peppermint herbal tea
- Bitter lemon or lemonade
- Lime cordial
- Ginger ale

- Sparkling mineral water with a slice of lemon or lime
- Fresh fruit juice diluted with sparkling mineral water
- Milkshakes made by blending skimmed milk with fresh fruits

Ginger

A great deal has been written about the effectiveness of ginger in treating different causes of nausea and vomiting. It can be taken in various forms; in drinks, cakes, biscuits and marmalade or in a capsule for a higher dosage. Ginger is believed to work in several ways. It increases the speed of digestion (which slows down naturally during pregnancy) and therefore minimises the likelihood of feeling or being sick. It is also believed to have a direct effect upon the part of the brain responsible for controlling nausea and vomiting, and it is one of the best food sources of zinc (the deficiency of which has been linked to morning sickness).

Zinc and the treatment of morning sickness

Zinc deficiency has already been linked to various types of depression, but in some cases it is also believed to cause morning sickness. Try to ensure that your diet includes zinc-rich foods such as shellfish and ginger. Many women have noticed a marked reduction in their sickness within a couple of weeks of taking a zinc supplement. If you do take a zinc supplement do not take it at the same time as the following food and drinks as they will actually prevent its absorption: chemical iron supplements, caffeine, milk, cheese, soya-based foods, celery, lemons, high-fibre foods such as wholemeal bread and bran.

Magnesium deficiency

As with zinc, a deficiency in the mineral magnesium has also been linked to feelings of nausea. Any deficiency can be corrected by a magnesium-rich diet (see the foods on page 110) or by taking milk of magnesia tablets, which soothe the stomach as well as raising magnesium levels.

Foods rich in magnesium

Spinach, broccoli, avocado, beans

Sunflower and pumpkin seeds

Cereals and wheatgerm

Nuts

Shrimps

Taking vitamin and mineral supplements

If you are suffering from nausea and vomiting during your pregnancy, and are simply unable to eat a diet rich in all the nutrients
your body requires, you may consider taking supplements instead.
By taking supplements you will at least have the reassurance that
you are meeting your body's requirements and, hopefully, within a
couple of weeks, you will notice some reduction in your sickness.
Look for a supplement that contains the following vitamins and
minerals:

Folic acid: 400mcg daily for at least one month before conception until 14 weeks pregnant

Vitamin A: try to avoid taking vitamin A supplement as it
can be toxic in large doses and has been linked to birth
defects

Vitamin B complex: containing at least the RDAs of vitamins
B1, B2, B3, B5, B6 and B12

Vitamin C: approx. 100mg daily

Vitamin E: 10mg daily

Calcium: approx. 200–300mg daily

Iron: 30mg daily (if you are anaemic you will require a higher
dosage)

Zinc: 15mg daily

Magnesium: 320mg daily (do not take at the same time as iron
supplement as it interferes with the body's absorption)

Eating patterns and morning sickness

For a lot of women pregnancy sickness is never solely confined to the morning. In the worst cases it can continue through the day and night. However, there are usually certain times when feelings of nausea are at their lowest. These are the times around which you should plan to eat. During the worst times (usually first thing in the morning) limit your intake to crackers and fluids and save the more nutritional snacks for when you are feeling at your best and are less likely to bring them back up.

Sleeping Problems

A common symptom of antenatal depression, and indeed pregnancy itself, is difficulty sleeping. Mental anxieties and physical discomfort as the baby grows can lead to many a sleepless night. This in turn leads to tiredness and increased feelings of anxiety. Although diet may not be the cause of this problem there are certain foods to avoid in the hours before you go to bed and certain foods that will actually encourage a good night's sleep.

Foods that can prevent sleep

- Sugary carbohydrates: sweets, chocolate, cakes
- Caffeine-loaded drinks: tea, coffee and cola
- Spicy foods
- Heavy meals late at night

Foods that encourage sleep

- Warm milk
- Bananas
- Wholemeal toast or sandwich

Diet and Postnatal Depression

Diet is just as important for the sufferer of postnatal depression. Many of the nutritional deficiencies that can be triggered by pregnancy are also likely to be present in the first few months after giving birth. Coupled with the exhaustion of sleepless nights and the general demands of a new-born baby, a healthy, well-balanced diet will ensure that the mother is receiving the maximum amount of energy and nutrition available. Not only will this eliminate any dietary causes of depression, but it will also provide the mother with a much-needed mental boost.

Nutritional deficiencies leading to depression

As with antenatal depression, deficiencies in iron, zinc and the B vitamins are all quite common in the weeks following the birth and are all known to cause feelings of exhaustion as well as despair. For advice on how to combat these deficiencies please see the previous section entitled 'Nutritional Deficiencies Caused by Pregnancy' (p. 103).

Restoring lost energy

When energy levels are low it is all too easy to become hooked on increasing amounts of caffeine and sugar. Nikki describes the weeks following the birth of her second child:

> 'It was a total blur. I have never felt so exhausted in all my life. I thought it had been bad enough after the birth of my first child, but nothing could have prepared me for having to look after a new baby, a toddler and a husband. I was a slave to Coca Cola and chocolate – if anybody had suggested healthy eating to me I would have probably bitten their head off. In those days caffeine was the only thing keeping me conscious, I'm sure of it.'

Although caffeine is a stimulant its effect is short term and it also interferes with the body's uptake of the vital minerals, iron and zinc. Deficiencies in these minerals are known to cause feelings of fatigue and depression so it is advisable to keep tea, coffee and cola consumption to a minimum, and then only between meals. Although sugary carbohydrates such as sweets and cakes provide an instant energy boost this is also very short-lived. Your blood sugar quickly returns to its previously low level, leaving you feeling even more tired. You then get caught in the trap of craving more and more sugar in order to maintain your energy levels. This in turn leads to weight gain and all the other negative feelings associated with 'bingeing'.

When eating for energy there are certain foods you should avoid and certain foods of which you should eat plenty.

Foods to avoid

Refined carbohydrates: white bread and bakery products, cakes, sweets

Sugar: avoid adding to drinks, cereal, etc.

Caffeine: tea, coffee, cola

Sweetened drinks: fizzy drinks and squashes sweetened with sugar

Excess bran: too much bran can interfere with the absorption of iron, zinc and magnesium

---

Foods for energy

Wholegrain cereals: Wholewheat pasta, brown rice, wholegrain breakfast cereals such as muesli, and the different types of wholegrain, wholemeal, rye and seeded bread all provide iron, B vitamins, vitamin E and much more fibre than the refined, white alternatives.

Nuts and seeds: Walnuts, hazel-nuts, Brazil nuts (avoid peanuts when pregnant or breast-feeding), sesame, sunflower and pumpkin seeds make a tasty snack on their own and are also a delicious topping for cereal or yoghurt and a tasty addition to various cake and biscuit recipes. Nuts provide an excellent source of protein, and both nuts and seeds contain large amounts of vitamins B complex and E and the essential minerals iron, zinc and potassium.

Pulses: Beans, lentils and tofu all make excellent alternative sources of protein to meat and provide additional fibre, B vitamins and minerals.

Fruit and vegetables: Aim to eat five portions of fresh fruit and vegetables every day (this can include one glass of fresh fruit juice). Fruit and vegetables are the best natural source of vitamin C. Bananas and baked potatoes are full of nutritional value, containing minerals and fibre as well as various vitamins.

Garlic: For centuries garlic has been used as a treatment for many different ailments. It is believed to increase energy levels and promote a general sense of well-being. Use it as a healthy alternative to salt for seasoning food.

Dried fruit: Apricots, prunes, raisins, dates and figs all provide an excellent source of minerals, especially iron, and provide a much better energy source than sweets or chocolate.

Eggs: As long as they are properly cooked, eggs are an excellent, all-round source of nutrients, containing iron, zinc and B vitamins as well as protein.

Poultry: Chicken and turkey provide a low-fat source of protein as well as vitamin B complex and iron.

Red meat: Lean cuts of beef, pork or lamb offer the best possible source of iron, zinc and B vitamins. Avoid frying to keep the fat content down.

Fish: All fish provide an excellent source of protein, but oily fish, particularly sardines, also contain iron and calcium.

Dairy products: Milk, yoghurt, fromage frais and cheese are all an excellent source of calcium, vital for the mother as well as the baby. By sticking to the low-fat, skimmed varieties you will obtain all the goodness of the calcium without an unhealthily high fat content.

Methods of cooking to increase energy

It is not just the food you eat, but the way you cook it that affects your energy levels.

Fruit and vegetables

Wherever possible fruit and vegetables should be eaten fresh and raw. Include plenty of salads, both fruit and vegetable, which are relatively quick and easy to prepare or can even be bought ready-made from the supermarket. When cooking vegetables use as little water as possible, and after cooking try adding this water to gravy or sauce so that none of the nutrients are lost.

Meat, poultry and fish

The key to cooking meat is to keep levels of fat as low as possible. Grilling, baking and poaching, therefore, should all be used as alternatives to frying. If frying, use a small amount of olive oil or sunflower oil in a wok.

Recipes and Meal Ideas for Energy and Nutrition

BREAKFAST

A good breakfast is important for all of us, but during pregnancy and the first few months after the birth it is absolutely vital. A high fibre, nutritious start to the day will provide you with the energy needed following the hours without food during the night. If you go without breakfast you are far more likely to snack on other, less nutritious, food mid-morning.

Toasted bananas and honey

2 slices of wholemeal bread
honey
1 tsp sesame seeds
sliced banana
glass of orange juice

Place slices of wholemeal bread under a moderate grill and toast on one side only. Remove bread from the grill and spread the untoasted side with honey. Sprinkle sesame seeds over each slice of bread. Top with sliced banana. Return to the grill for a few minutes until golden brown. Serve with a glass of orange juice.

Fruit smoothies

Smoothies can be made with any combination of fruit. By adding as many different fruits as possible they make an ideal way of meeting the desired five portions a day. They can be made the night before in larger quantities in order to save time in the morning and can be consumed throughout the day.

10 strawberries (with the stalks removed)
2 kiwi fruit (peeled and sliced)
200ml (1/3 pint) milk
2 slices buttered, wholemeal toast

Place strawberries and kiwi fruit in a blender. Blend for about a minute, until all lumps are gone. Add milk and blend for another minute. Pour into a tall glass and serve with buttered, wholemeal toast.

Muesli

You can make your own muesli from scratch, but to save time buy it ready made from a supermarket and add your own choice of nuts, seeds and dried fruits.

> *1 tsp sesame seeds*
> *1 tbsp sunflower seeds*
> *bowl unsweetened muesli*
> *chopped, dried apricots*
> *skimmed milk*
> *glass of orange juice*

Add sesame seeds and sunflower seeds to a bowl of unsweetened muesli. Add apricots and any other dried fruit you like and mix well. Serve with skimmed milk and an accompanying glass of orange juice.

Porridge

Porridge is suitably bland for the sufferer of morning sickness and extra nutrients can easily be added.

Make up some porridge with skimmed milk. Pick one of the following additions:
> *1 tbsp sesame seeds and a sprinkling of cinnamon*
> *ginger marmalade*
> *lemon juice*
> *chopped dates and walnuts*
> *sliced banana*
> *grated apple and raisins*

Serve with a glass of fruit juice and a piece of fresh fruit.

Scrambled eggs

Scrambled eggs contain a wide range of nutrients. If you have the time add chopped vegetables for extra vitamins.

half a finely chopped onion
finely chopped green pepper
olive or sunflower oil
2 eggs
dash of milk
salt and pepper
toasted wholemeal muffin or toast
banana
glass of fruit juice

Sauté onion and/or green pepper in olive or sunflower oil. Beat eggs with a dash of milk and salt and pepper to taste. Add to the onion and pepper and cook until well scrambled. Serve on muffin or toast with a banana and a glass of fruit juice.

Strawberry and kiwi fruit yoghurt

If you find natural yoghurt a bit sour on its own add your own choice of fresh or dried fruits to sweeten it up.

sliced strawberries
sliced kiwi fruits
organic yoghurt
chopped, roasted hazelnuts
2 slices wholemeal toast
lemon herbal tea

Place sliced strawberries and kiwi fruits in a bowl. Cover with natural, organic yoghurt. Sprinkle chopped, roasted hazelnuts on top. Serve with wholemeal toast and lemon herbal tea.

Yoghurt crunch

1 serving of crunchy, muesli-type cereal
1 tbsp sesame seeds
1 tbsp sunflower seeds
1 tbsp chopped nuts
1 tbsp dried apricots
natural yogurt
toast
fruit juice

Take a normal serving of crunchy, muesli-type cereal. Add to the cereal the sesame seeds, sunflower seeds, chopped nuts and dried apricots. Spoon over as much natural yoghurt as you require. Serve with toast and fruit juice.

Fresh fruit salad

Fruit salad can be made in large quantities and stored in the fridge to save time in the morning. If you are feeling down or suffering from morning sickness try to pick sharp-tasting, citrus fruits to wake up the taste buds and help alleviate feelings of nausea.

chunks of fresh pineapple
grapes
kiwi fruit
orange
grapefruit
fruit juice or natural yoghurt
wholemeal toast or muffin
herbal tea

Prepare chunks of fruit in a bowl. Top with fruit juice or natural yoghurt. Serve with wholemeal toast or muffin and herbal tea.

Bacon and cheese muffin

2 rashers of bacon
1 wholemeal muffin
grated cheese
grilled tomato
glass of fruit juice

Grill bacon and toast wholemeal muffin. Place one rasher of bacon on each half of the muffin. Sprinkle some grated cheese over the top of each and return to the grill briefly for cheese to turn golden brown. Serve with a grilled tomato and a glass of fruit juice.

Healthy breakfast in a rush

If time is at a premium try any two of the following for a quick nutritious breakfast:

Any wholegrain, high-fibre breakfast cereal with extra sesame
    seeds, chopped dried apricots and skimmed milk
Wholemeal toast or muffin with Marmite spread
A banana
A glass of fresh orange juice
Natural yoghurt with honey, sesame seeds and chopped nuts

LUNCH AND LIGHT MEALS

A healthy, well-balanced lunch will provide you with the energy you need to get through the afternoon. If you are suffering from morning sickness, lunch could well be your first proper meal of the day, so it is even more important that you consume as many nutrients as possible. Most of these meal ideas can be prepared in advance and taken in to work as a healthy alternative to fish and chips from the canteen. Each meal should be accompanied by a glass of fruit juice and at least one piece of fresh fruit.

Stuffed pitta bread

Wholemeal pitta bread offers a tasty alternative to ordinary bread. Warm under a moderate grill and stuff with one of the following fillings:

Tuna salad
tin of tuna
2 chopped, hard-boiled eggs
3 finely chopped spring onions
1 large, chopped tomato
mayonnaise
ground black pepper

Drain tin of tuna and separate into flakes in a bowl. Add eggs, spring onions and tomato. Stir together and add mayonnaise and ground black pepper to taste. This makes enough for two pittas, so any extra can be stored in the refrigerator for later.

Lemon chicken and hummus
1 chicken breast fillet
2 tbsp olive oil
juice of 1 lemon
1 tsp dried lemon grass
hummus

Cut chicken breast fillet into thin strips. In a bowl mix together olive oil, lemon juice and lemon grass. Add the chicken strips to the lemon mixture and make sure each piece is well coated. Cover the bowl and leave to marinate in the refrigerator for at least an hour. Place the chicken in the bottom of the grill pan and cook under a moderate heat for 10–15 minutes until chicken is cooked right through. Spread the inside of a warmed pitta bread with hummus and add the lemon chicken.

Swiss cheese and ham
Swiss cheese
ham
tomato
watercress

Fill a warm pitta bread with slices of Swiss cheese, ham, tomato and watercress.

Sardines on toast

Sardines are one of the best sources of iron and calcium available. Aim to have at least two servings every week.

2 slices wholemeal bread
120g (5oz) tin sardines
thin slices of tomato
mixed herbs

Place wholemeal bread under the grill and toast on one side. Drain sardines and mash with a fork. Spread the sardines on the untoasted side of the bread, top with tomato and sprinkle mixed herbs over the top. Return to the grill until tomatoes begin to brown.

Vegetable soup

Vegetable soup is an excellent source of vitamins and can be made in large quantities and stored in the fridge.

1 tbsp olive oil
1 finely chopped onion
1 crushed clove garlic
1 x 2.5cm (1in) piece of fresh root ginger, finely chopped and
*   peeled*
1 tin chopped tomatoes
1.2l (2 pints) vegetable stock
1 green pepper
250g (9oz) mushrooms
2 leeks
wholemeal bread

Heat the olive oil in the bottom of a large saucepan. Add the onion to the oil and cook gently for about 5 minutes. Stir in the garlic, root ginger and tomatoes. Cook over a low heat for a further 5 minutes. Add vegetable stock and vegetables. Bring to the boil, then simmer on a low heat for about an hour. Serve with crusty wholemeal bread.

Avocado salad

1 avocado pear
lemon juice
tinned salmon
finely chopped spring onions
sliced tomatoes
watercress
crusty wholegrain roll or bread

Cut the avocado pear in half and remove the stone. Sprinkle the flesh with lemon juice (this prevents discolouring as well as adding flavour). Fill each half with tinned salmon mixed with spring onions. Serve with the tomatoes on a bed of watercress and the roll or bread.

Vegetable risotto

225g (8oz) brown rice
900ml (1¹/2 pints) vegetable stock
1 tbsp olive or sunflower oil
1 chopped onion
1 green and 1 red pepper, chopped
250g (9oz) sliced mushrooms
2 sliced leeks
25g (1oz) pumpkin seeds

Place brown rice in a large saucepan. Add vegetable stock and bring to the boil. Then simmer gently over a low heat for about 30 minutes until all the liquid has been absorbed by the rice. While the rice is cooking heat olive or sunflower oil in a large frying pan or wok. Gently fry onion for about 3–4 minutes until softened. Add peppers, mushrooms and leeks. Continue cooking over a gentle heat for a further 5–10 minutes. When the rice is cooked drain off any excess vegetable stock and stir into the vegetables. Sprinkle pumpkin seeds over the top and serve.

Healthy lunch in a rush

We do not always have the time to cook a meal in the middle of the day so here are some nutritious lunchtime ideas for meals on the go:

> Add watercress and use wholemeal bread when making sandwiches to increase your iron intake.
> Buy ready-prepared salads from the supermarket.
> Make sure your lunchtime drink is high in vitamin C, such as orange or blackcurrant juice, so that your body will absorb the iron in your diet.
> Replace crisps with a mixture of nuts and/or dried fruit.
> Baked potatoes
> Baked beans on toast
> Health food bars and fresh fruit as an alternative to cakes or sweets

MAIN MEALS

A healthy main meal will provide a welcome energy boost after a busy, tiring day. It will also ensure that your sleep will not be disrupted by indigestion or high blood-sugar levels.

Tuna fishcakes

> 2 tins tuna, drained and flaked
> 1 onion, finely chopped
> 1 tbsp fresh chopped parsley
> a handful breadcrumbs (2 slices bread)
> juice of 1 lemon
> 2 egg yolks
> olive oil
> watercress
> lemon wedges

Mix together tuna, onion, parsley and breadcrumbs. Add to this mixture the lemon juice and egg yolks. Stir well until mixture is combined. Mould into four cakes and fry in olive oil over a moderate heat for about 5 minutes each side until golden brown. Serve with a pasta salad and garnish with watercress and lemon wedges, or with melted cheese in a wholegrain roll.

Grilled sardines

fresh sardines
olive oil
lemon juice
dried lemon grass

Marinate fresh sardines in a mixture of olive oil, lemon juice and lemon grass. Grill under a moderate heat for 7–8 minutes each side, until fish are cooked through and crispy on the outside. Serve with a baked potato, pasta salad or brown rice.

Meatloaf

1 onion
1 green pepper, finely chopped
2 slices bread made into crumbs
1 tsp chopped parsley
1 tsp Worcester sauce
1 beaten egg
1/4 cup water
3 tbsp tomato purée
450g (1lb) lean minced beef

In a large mixing bowl place onion, green pepper, breadcrumbs; chopped parsley, Worcester sauce, beaten egg, water and tomato purée. Mix well. Add minced beef and combine with the rest of the mixture. Place in a greased, lined loaf tin and bake for 1 hour at 180°C (350°F, Gas mark 4) or until brown on top. Serve in slices with gravy, baked potato and vegetables of your choice.

Chicken with bacon and cheese

1 chicken breast fillet
thin slices of Cheddar cheese
2 rashers bacon

Place chicken breast fillet on a baking tray. Cover with Cheddar cheese and top with bacon. Bake for about 30 minutes at 200°C (400°F, Gas mark 6). Serve with a watercress and tomato salad and a baked potato or crusty wholemeal bread.

Vegetable pasta sauce

1 tbsp olive oil
1 finely chopped onion
1 chopped green, red or yellow pepper
250g (9oz) chopped mushrooms
2 sliced courgettes
1 tin chopped tomatoes
1 tbsp tomato purée
mixed herbs
pasta
grated cheese

Heat olive oil in a large frying pan or wok. Add onion and cook gently for about 5 minutes. Add pepper, mushrooms and courgettes and stir fry for about 10 minutes until vegetables are cooked. Add tomatoes, tomato purée and a sprinkling of mixed herbs. Simmer for a further 10 minutes. Serve with pasta and top with grated cheese.

Roasted vegetables

1 yellow pepper
1 green pepper
2 onions
2 courgettes
1 large aubergine
250g (9oz) mushrooms
2 large tomatoes
dried rosemary
black pepper

Chop the vegetables into large chunks. Place the vegetables in a lightly oiled roasting tin and brush with olive oil. Sprinkle with dried rosemary and black pepper. Roast for 25 minutes at 220°C (425°F, Gas mark 7), turning half way through. Serve as a tasty accompaniment to chicken or fish.

Shortcuts to healthy main meals
- Prepacked stir-fry vegetables
- Baked potatoes instead of chips
- Grill or bake instead of frying
- Always have a vegetable or salad accompaniment
- Replace sugary desserts with a piece of fruit or a yoghurt.

HEALTHY SNACKS

When you are tired and run down, nutritious snacks become an important part of the diet, providing a valuable energy boost in between meals. If you are suffering from chronic morning sickness your diet may consist solely of snacks so it is vital they have a high nutritional value. Try some of the following ideas as a healthy alternative to crisps and sweets:

Fruity flapjacks

These flapjacks keep very well if stored in an airtight container, so you could make double the quantity to save on cooking time. They are an excellent source of energy, vitamins and minerals.

100g (4oz) margarine
75g (3oz) golden syrup
50g (2oz) brown sugar
200g (8oz) rolled oats
25g (1oz) sesame seeds
25g (1oz) sunflower seeds
50g (2oz) raisins or chopped dried apricots

Melt the margarine with the golden syrup and brown sugar over a low to moderate heat. Remove from heat and stir in the rolled oats, sesame seeds, sunflower seeds and raisins or apricots. Turn into a greased shallow 20-cm (8-in) square tin and flatten down with a palette knife. Bake in a preheated oven at 180°C (350°F, Gas mark 4) for 25–30 minutes until golden brown. Cool in tin for 2 minutes, then cut into fingers. Allow to cool completely before removing from tin.

Banana and walnut loaf

Fruit loaves make an excellent healthy alternative to sugary cakes. Experiment with different fruits such as dried apricots or dates.

100g (4oz) sunflower margarine
50g (4oz) soft brown sugar
2 large eggs
3 large mashed bananas
200g (8oz) plain wholemeal flour
1 tsp baking powder
1/2 tsp ground cinnamon
75g (3oz) chopped walnuts

Preheat oven to 180°C (350°F, Gas mark 4) and grease and line a 900g (2lb) loaf tin. Cream the margarine with the sugar until light and fluffy. Beat in eggs, one at a time. Beat in bananas. Fold in flour, baking powder, cinnamon and walnuts. Pour into the loaf tin and bake for 1–1¼ hours until a skewer inserted into the middle of the loaf comes out clean. Leave to cool in the tin for 5 minutes then turn out onto a wire cooling rack. As an alternative to banana use 50g (2oz) of chopped ready-to-eat dried apricots and 1 large apple, grated.

Ginger biscuits

An excellent source of zinc; try these if you are suffering from morning sickness.

50g (2oz) sunflower margarine
4 tbsp golden syrup
50g (2oz) soft brown sugar
150g (6oz) wholewheat flour
1 tsp ground ginger
1 tsp grated root ginger
1 tbsp chopped preserved ginger

Pre-heat oven to 190°C (375°F, Gas mark 5) and grease two baking sheets. Melt the margarine, golden syrup and sugar over a low to moderate heat. Remove from heat and stir in the flour, ground ginger, root ginger and preserved ginger. Mix to a smooth paste. Roll into balls the size of a walnut and place on greased baking sheet spaced well apart. Bake for 15–20 minutes. Leave on sheet for 1 minute before removing to a wire cooling rack.

Quick and easy wholemeal soda bread

This bread is full of the essential B vitamins and minerals and an excellent source of fibre. It is easy to make and requires no kneading.

450g (1lb) wholemeal bread flour
50g (2oz) bran
50g (2oz) wheatgerm
1 tsp salt
1 tsp sugar
1 tsp bicarbonate of soda
600ml (1 pint) milk

Pre-heat oven to 190°C (375°F, Gas mark 5) and grease and line a 900g (2lb) loaf tin. In a large bowl, mix together the flour, bran, wheatgerm, salt, sugar and bicarbonate of soda. Slowly add the milk to the mixture, stirring well until it forms a dough (if mixture is too dry continue slowly adding small amounts of milk, stirring continuously). Place dough in loaf tin and press down evenly with a fork until mixture is level. Bake for 50 minutes, until golden brown on top. Leave in tin to cool for 5 minutes then turn out on to a wire cooling rack.

Halvah

If you have a sweet tooth halvah makes a nutritious alternative to sweets and chocolate. It is packed full of sesame seeds (an excellent source of zinc and calcium). Halvah can be bought ready-made in tubs from the supermarket or health food store, but it is very easy to make yourself.

> *125g (5oz) sesame seeds*
> *2 tsp fairly solid honey*

Take the sesame seeds and remove 1 tablespoon full. Grind the larger amount of sesame seeds into a powder. Stir in the honey until mixture forms a thick paste. Roll into balls and coat with the remaining, unground sesame seeds.

Cigarettes

Mothers are constantly warned about the adverse effects of their drinking and smoking upon their baby, and this is not without reason. Both alcohol and the carbon monoxide present in cigarettes are poisons which, if consumed by the pregnant mother, will be directly transmitted to the foetus. Even after the birth there are known health risks for a baby living in a smoky environment, including increased risk of cot death and breathing complications such as asthma. However, for the sufferer of antenatal or postnatal depression sometimes a sneaky puff on a cigarette or the odd glass of wine seems like the only thing preventing you from a complete mental breakdown. In a similar way to comfort eating it doesn't take long before the source of consolation becomes the source of distress, as Natalie discovered during her first pregnancy:

> *'I had always been a heavy drinker and smoker. I wasn't an alcoholic or anything but I was really into clubbing, and*

cigarettes and alcohol were a big part of my lifestyle. The minute I discovered I was pregnant I stopped – to be honest it wasn't that difficult at first – my morning sickness meant that I couldn't bear the smell of cigarette smoke and I didn't really fancy a drink either. Things started to go wrong at about the fourth month. My sickness disappeared, but mentally I became a bit of a wreck. I was the first one from my group of friends to get pregnant and at first it was great; everybody made a big fuss of me. But after the fuss died down I was left at home while they carried on going out enjoying themselves. My relationship hit the rocks too, I had thought that my pregnancy would bring us closer together and that the problems we had been having would disappear, but they just seemed to get worse. I started to panic – I don't think I was really ready for the responsibility of being a mum. One day I was walking down the street and a man in front of me lit up a cigarette. Instead of making me feel sick it smelt lovely. I went straight to the nearest newsagent and bought a packet of ten. I must have spent hours just staring at them before I actually smoked one. I knew all about the dangers but I couldn't take the stress anymore. I was used to lighting up at the first sign of pressure. Afterwards I felt terrible – I pictured my baby floating around inside me in a cloud of smoke – but I didn't know how I was going to get through my pregnancy without cigarettes. Most days I smoked fewer than five, but when things got really bad – the days I just couldn't stop crying – I would smoke up to 20. It was like a vicious circle. The more I smoked the worse I felt about what I might be doing to my baby, but the worse I felt the more I wanted a cigarette.'

Everyone agrees that it is better not to smoke at all during pregnancy, but in cases of antenatal depression this is not always possible. If stress and anxiety have you reaching for a cigarette you must bear in mind the health risks to your child and take the steps necessary to reduce these risks.

The risks of smoking to the baby

- **Death:** Smoking over ten cigarettes a day will increase the risk to your baby of miscarriage, stillbirth and cot death, so you should make every possible effort to keep below this figure.
- **Low birth weight:** If you manage to stop smoking by half way through your pregnancy or cut right down to below five a day, you will drastically reduce the chances of your baby having a low birth weight.
- **Congenital deformities:** Any smoking during pregnancy carries the risk of some form of congenital deformity to the baby, such as a cleft palate or a hare lip.

Tips for reducing the risks to your child

- Cut down to fewer than ten cigarettes a day or preferably fewer than five
- Have your first cigarette as late in the day as possible
- Smoke the lowest tar cigarette possible
- Only smoke the first half of the cigarette, as there is far more tar and nicotine in the bottom half
- Never smoke roll-ups, always use a filter
- Try to give up completely or cut right down before week 20 of your pregnancy
- Use relaxation techniques or sugar-free chewing gum as an alternative stress reliever
- Take extra zinc, vitamins B6, B12 and C either in your diet or in supplement form, as smoking will deplete your body of these nutrients

Alcohol

As with smoking and binge eating, alcohol is a common crutch for the sufferer of depression. The irony is that although drinking may give you a temporary buzz, alcohol is actually a depressant and is far more likely to make you feel worse in the long run. Experts seem to disagree upon the damage that alcohol can cause to the unborn child, with some doctors saying that there is no harm in one or two drinks a day and others advising that alcohol should be totally avoided throughout the pregnancy. Consuming more than two alcoholic drinks a day has been linked to facial abnormalities, heart defects and lower than average intelligence and birthweight in the baby. Once again, sufferers of antenatal and postnatal depression can become caught up in a cycle of turning to drink as a stress reliever only for it to become a source of guilt over the potential damage they may be doing their child. Kay started drinking heavily during her battle with postnatal depression after the birth of her son, Josh:

'I had quite a stressful pregnancy, what with various health scares and the general anxieties of becoming a mum. On more than one occasion I longed for a nice cold vodka and tonic, but I was very good and didn't touch a drop. I was far too worried about the health of my baby anyway – the last thing I wanted to do was increase the risks of something going wrong. However, once I had given birth I had real problems breast-feeding and I think this prevented me from bonding properly with Josh. I became really depressed. I wasn't anxious like before – it was just like this big, black cloud hanging over me. One day, when Josh was about four weeks old, I went out for a drink with a friend. It had been so long since I had drunk alcohol I only had two and I was under the table. It was a lovely, warm feeling and I remember coming home and sinking into bed without a care in the world. Of course it was a different story two hours later when I had to get up for the night feed – my head was thumping and I felt so lousy I made myself another drink. Before I knew it I was drinking every day, using the excuse that it was for medicinal purposes, to help me to relax and sleep. It wasn't hard to keep my drinking hidden as my husband was out at work all day and *he was asleep when I did the night feeds. If I seemed a bit absent-minded or out of it he put it down to tiredness or depression. In the end it took a potential tragedy for me to sort myself out and seek help. I'd put Josh down on the bedroom floor to play and I was so drunk I just dozed off on the bed. I woke up later and he'd disappeared. I staggered out on to the landing and he'd managed to roll himself right to the very edge of the stairs. I have never been so terrified in all my life – he could have been seriously injured or even killed and I was lying in a drunken stupor on the bed. This is what prompted me to seek help from my doctor for my postnatal depression. However bad I felt or however hard I found it to bond with my son I could never have lived with myself if anything bad had happened to him.'*

Tips to help control your drinking

- Limit your alcohol consumption to no more than 1 unit a day.
- Try not to drink every day of the week; aim to limit it to just once or twice.
- Drink low alcohol alternatives rather than strong spirits, extra strength beer or lager.
- Eat a healthy diet to decrease your desire to drink.
- If you feel your drinking is spiralling out of control do not be afraid to seek help. Phone Alcoholics Anonymous (see page 171) for helpful advice and support; you don't have to give your real name and no one will judge you unfit to be a mother. On the contrary, by seeking help you will be showing responsibility towards your child.

Chapter 8
Exercise and Relaxation Techniques

Pregnancy and the birth of a new child provide the perfect excuses not to exercise. *'What's the point? I'm going to look like the back of a bus anyway'*, and *'When the hell am I supposed to find the time?'* were two of my personal favourites. If you are suffering from antenatal or postnatal depression you would probably much rather pig out than work out, but exercise and relaxation do provide important psychological as well as physical gains. Regular exercise will actually increase your energy levels and stamina, release feel-good chemicals in the brain and improve your physical appearance. Relaxation techniques teach you to deal more effectively with stress and anxiety and will aid sleep. As with diet, exercise alone will not cure your depression, but it is an extremely effective way of regaining control of your life and taking that first important step back to happiness.

Exercise and Antenatal Depression

There are several ways in which regular exercise and relaxation can help the sufferer of antenatal depression:

- **Improving self-confidence.** We have seen how pregnancy can destroy self confidence and lead to feelings of depression. Exercise is a very effective way of regaining self-esteem, by giving you pride in your appearance and the knowledge that after the birth you will get back to your normal figure much quicker.

- **Preparing for the birth.** Antenatal depression often manifests itself in a chronic fear of the birth itself. By following a specific exercise and relaxation plan you will be able to prepare yourself both physically and mentally for the labour, and hopefully overcome some of your fears.

- **Managing stress and anxiety.** As a sufferer of antenatal depression your pregnancy is likely to be fraught with stress and anxiety. By learning different relaxation and breathing techniques you will be able to alleviate stress quickly and effectively, minimising any effect upon your baby. (The techniques will also prove invaluable during contractions.)

Before you start

The type of exercise you do depends very much upon your own level of fitness and of course your pregnancy. If you were already regularly exercising and are having a complication-free pregnancy you should have no problem in following a programme of gentle exercise. If, however, you have not been exercising prior to pregnancy, or have a history of miscarriage or other physical complications, you should consult your doctor before undertaking any form of exercise, particularly in the first three months. During the first trimester the pregnancy is establishing itself and this is known to be the most precarious time. It is therefore vital that you do not overdo it. Listen to your body, and if at any time during exercising you feel pain or faint, stop immediately. After the fourteenth week of pregnancy you should feel a new lease of life as your body adapts to the physical and hormonal changes and your energy levels rise again. If you are feeling depressed, this is an ideal time to start some form of exercise, in preparation mentally and physically for the birth. In the last trimester you will be growing larger and some exercises will become increasingly uncomfortable and awkward to do. You should adapt your exercises accordingly, but by no means stop altogether, as in the run up to the birth you will probably benefit from them more than ever.

What kind of exercise?

Walking and swimming are both ideal forms of gentle exercise during pregnancy. If you are not used to exercising, simply try walking more – aim for at least 20 minutes a day. Even in the winter you cannot beat fresh air for waking up the system and clearing out the cobwebs. Walking is also extremely therapeutic if you have a lot on your mind and need time to gather your thoughts. Swimming is an excellent all-round form of exercise and as long as you don't overdo it there is no reason why you cannot continue swimming right up until the birth. Dancing to up-tempo music is another good exercise for providing an instant mental boost, as long as you are not over-ambitious – break-dancing around your living room should be avoided at all costs.

Yoga

By far the most effective form of exercise in the treatment of ante-natal depression is yoga. This is because yoga encourages both physical and mental well-being, by incorporating gentle stretching with breathing, meditation and relaxation techniques.

The physical benefits of yoga during pregnancy

- It will help keep weight gain down.
- It helps to prevent stretch marks.
- It strengthens the back, preventing the aches and pains normally associated with pregnancy.
- It improves posture.
- It encourages more rapid recovery of muscle tone after the birth.

The mental benefits of yoga during pregnancy

- Through meditation you are taught to focus on the joy of creating a new life rather than the more negative aspects on which you may have been dwelling.
- By picturing the baby moving with you during your exercises you are encouraged to bond with your child before the birth.
- By teaching you to live in the present and creating deep resources of inner strength, yoga can help to conquer any fear of the birth itself.

- The main focus is on you and your body rather than the birth, therefore building self-esteem.
- Yoga teaches you to visualise energy as warmth, light or power. This is incorporated into the breathing techniques of each exercise. In this way you learn how to increase your own energy levels and conquer the feelings of lethargy associated with depression.

There are many yoga classes now available for pregnant women. Contact the British Wheel of Yoga for details of your local yoga instructor (see Useful Addresses section of this book on page 171 for further information). Alternatively, try the following programme of yoga exercises (or asanas) at home. Remember to be especially careful during your first trimester and only take each stretch as far as is comfortable.

Tips before you begin

- Stop if you feel any pain or become light-headed.
- Never practise yoga straight after eating – leave at least one hour after a light snack and two hours after a meal.
- Practise yoga away from any distractions, such as a noisy television or a laughing husband.
- Wear loose clothes and have bare feet.
- Use a mat or folded blanket on the floor beneath you.
- Have a chair handy and some space by an empty wall for support.
- Have a blanket or extra clothing for the warm-up and relaxation sections.
- Have a couple of cushions or pillows for comfort.
- Avoid lying flat on your back after week 30 of your pregnancy; instead lie on your side, using a cushion or pillow between your knees.
- Remember to follow the breathing instructions, and as you perform each exercise picture your baby moving with you.

Complete Yoga Routine

Centre yourself and relax

- Lie flat on your back on a mat or blanket. In later months it will be more comfortable to lie in the modified abdominal Corpse Position *(see illustration 1)*. Use cushions for support under your head, neck or leg as required.

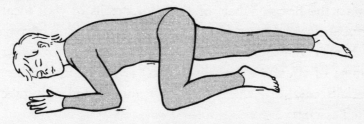

Illustration 1. *The modified abdominal Corpse Position*

- Let your legs relax apart and place your hands just above your waist, with your elbows resting on the floor.
- Focus on your breathing. As you take a deep breath in through your nose feel your hands rising with your abdomen and as you breathe out slowly, feel your hands sink back down.
- Count slowly in your head as you breathe in and out, making sure that each inhalation is the same length as each exhalation.
- Feel your whole body start to relax and focus your thoughts entirely upon your breathing, in and out through the nose.
- When you feel completely relaxed you are ready to move on to the warm-up section.

Warming up

Over-arm stretches

This exercise is a perfect way to wake the body up slowly. It should be performed as if in slow motion and it should never be forced.

- Lying flat on your back, check that your head and spine are aligned and then slowly stretch your arms over your head, taking a deep breath in through your nose.

- Remain in this position and gently push away with your feet so that your whole body is stretching *(see illustration 2)*.

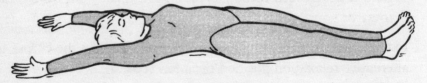

Illustration 2. *The over-arm stretch*

- Slowly return your arms to the floor by your sides, exhaling deeply.
- Repeat four times, remembering to breathe correctly. Try not to over stretch. Each movement should be slow and gentle.

The upturned Beetle

This exercise gently opens out the spine, easing out any tension, particularly in the lower back.

- Lie on your back and tuck your chin in slightly to extend your neck.
- Bend your knees and bring them up towards your chest.
- Place one hand on each of your knees and feel the whole length of your spine from your neck down to your tailbone making contact with the floor.
- Breathing in through the nose, slowly tilt your knees over to the right as you turn your head to the left and feel a gentle twist in the waist *(see illustration 3)*.
- Breathing out, return to the centre.

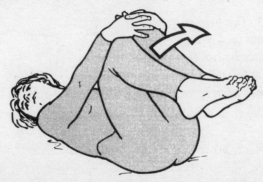

Illustration 3. *The upturned Beetle*

- Repeat this exercise to the other side and continue to rock gently from side-to-side until you have completed four on each side.
- Return to the centre and breathing in, gently lift your head towards your knees.

Extend your legs, relax your arms down and lie in the corpse or alternative relaxation position for a few seconds.

The pelvic lift

This exercise provides another excellent stretch for the spine, easing back pain and strengthening the uterus.

- On all fours, check that your hands are directly beneath your shoulders and your knees are directly beneath your hips.
- Exhale deeply through your nose and arch your spine upwards; feel your stomach being pulled inwards. Tuck your head in between your shoulders (see illustration 4).

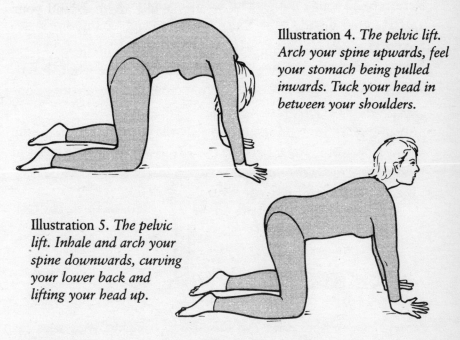

Illustration 4. *The pelvic lift. Arch your spine upwards, feel your stomach being pulled inwards. Tuck your head in between your shoulders.*

Illustration 5. *The pelvic lift. Inhale and arch your spine downwards, curving your lower back and lifting your head up.*

- Inhale and arch your spine downwards, curving your lower back and lifting your head up, looking up towards the ceiling (see illustration 5).

- Repeat slowly four times, remembering to breathe correctly through your nose.

Sink down on to your knees, rest your forehead on the ground, relax into the Child's Pose *(see illustration 8)* or its variation and stay there for a few seconds.

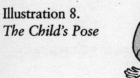
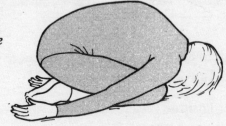

Illustration 8.
The Child's Pose

The Cat

This pose keeps your lower back supple and strengthens the legs.

- Return to all fours, inhale, and lift your right leg up behind you with the knee slightly bent. Raise your head and look up towards the ceiling.
- Slowly straighten out the raised leg and feel the stretch down your back *(see illustration 6)*.

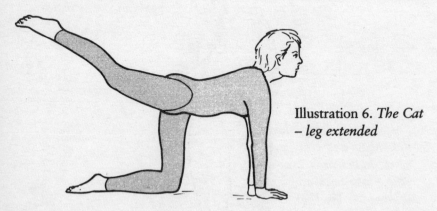

Illustration 6. *The Cat – leg extended*

- Slowly exhale and bend the raised leg, bringing your toes in towards your head.
- Lower your head and leg at the same time and try to bring your knee in towards your forehead *(see illustration 7)*.

Illustration 7. *The Cat – bring the knee in towards the forehead.*

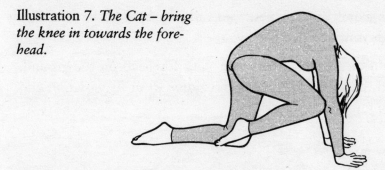

- Return your knee to the floor and repeat four times on each side.
- Relax in the Child's Pose *(see illustration 8)*.

Breathing in Prayer Position

An excellent stretch for the top half of the body, this position increases the flow of energy.

- Sit in a comfortable position, either cross-legged or legs slightly bent in front of you.
- Bring your hands in front of your chest in Prayer Position *(see illustration 9)*.

Illustration 9. *Breathing in Prayer Position*

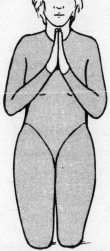

- Inhale deeply through your nose as you raise your hands, still pressed together, straight up past your head and feel the top half of your body stretching upwards.

- Exhale and let your arms open out to the sides as your hands return down to the floor.
- Breathe in as your arms slowly reach out to the sides. Stretch upwards as your hands meet again over your head.
- Exhale as you bring your joined hands back to the Prayer Position in front of your chest.

The seated spinal twist

This pose improves flexibility in the spine and the waist.

- Sit cross-legged and place your left hand on your right knee and your right hand flat on the floor behind you.
- Inhale and twist your body gently to the right, looking over your right shoulder (see illustration 10).

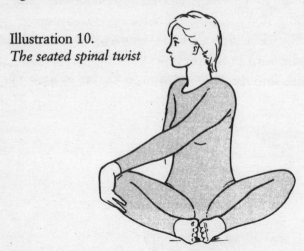

Illustration 10.
The seated spinal twist

- Hold this position, breathing deeply through your nose.
- Repeat to the other side.

Standing stretches

Basic standing stretch

Standing stretches are excellent for all-over strength and posture.

- Stand up straight with legs slightly apart and knees slightly bent.
- Slowly inhale and raise your right hand up towards the ceiling as you bend your left knee. Look up towards the raised hand.

- Exhale and return to starting position. Repeat four times on each side.

Relax by flopping forwards at the waist and letting your head hang down between your bent legs.

The Tree

This position improves balance both physically and mentally, by developing your power of concentration and focusing your mind.

- Stand up still and straight. Imagine that there is a piece of string attached to the top of your head, pulling you upright.
- Draw your right foot slowly up the inside of your left calf, turning your knee outwards. If you feel steady bring your hands into the Prayer Position in front of your chest. Maintain this pose for a while, breathing slowly and steadily through your nose.
- If you are wobbly use a chair on your right side. Place your right foot on the chair, turn both foot and knee out to the side and bring your hands into the Prayer Position *(see illustration 11).*

Illustration 11.
The Tree – with chair

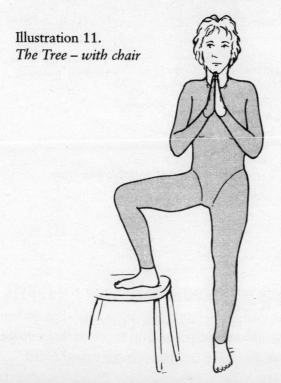

- With your right hand bring your right foot up to the inside of your left thigh. Press the sole of your foot into your thigh.
- When you are balanced bring your hands into the Prayer Position and raise them straight up above your head *(see illustration 12)*. Hold the pose for as long as you feel comfortable. If you start wobbling return to standing position.
- Repeat on the other side of the body.

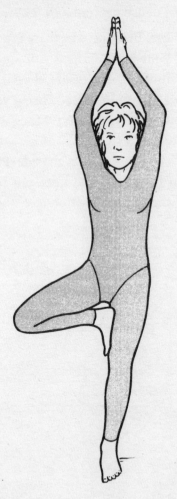

Illustration 12. *The Tree – fully extended, without chair*

Relax by flopping forwards at the waist and let your head hang down between your bent legs.

Modified stretches

The modified shoulderstand

The shoulderstand takes the strain off your legs and back, improving circulation. Do not remove your legs from the wall until you have practised this position several times.

- Lie on your back next to a wall, with your buttocks pressed against the wall and your legs stretched up it.
- Press into the wall with your feet, raising your back enough to place your hands underneath for support.
- Walk your feet upwards until your legs are straight.
- When your legs are straight slowly lift one leg at a time away from the wall *(see illustration 13).*

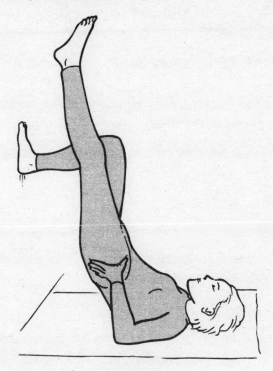

Illustration 13. *The modified shoulderstand*

The modified Plough

As a follow-up pose to the modified shoulderstand, the Plough provides an excellent stretch for the lower back.

- From the modified shoulderstand slowly allow your legs to drop down to rest on a chair behind you. Push your heels backwards and breath deeply *(see illustration 14)*.

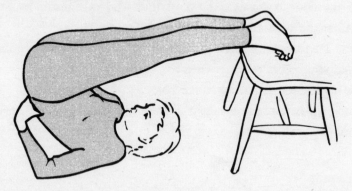

Illustration 14. *The modified Plough*

- Push your legs back to the wall one at a time and slowly lower your back down to the floor.

Rest in the corpse position *(see illustration 1)* or variation.

Cool down

Wall stretches

These exercises are an excellent way both to cool down and to prepare the pelvis for the birth itself.

The wall Butterfly

- Lie with your buttocks and feet pressed against the wall. Bring the soles of your feet together and allow your knees to drop open.
- Press your knees down and towards the wall with your hands *(see illustration 15)*.
- Relax and breathe slowly and rhythmically.

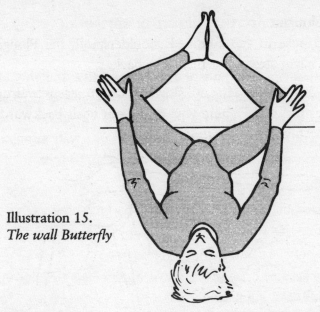

Illustration 15.
The wall Butterfly

Wall squats

- Lying with your buttocks pressed against the wall, separate your feet wide apart and press against the wall.
- Gently pull your knees out and down with your hands (*see illustration 16*).
- Relax and focus once more on your breathing.

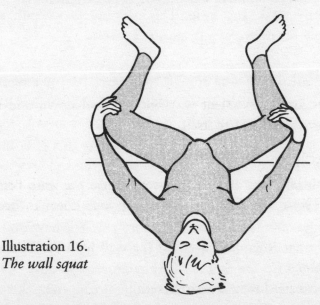

Illustration 16.
The wall squat

Relaxation technique for the sufferer of antenatal depression

The final relaxation is a vital part of any yoga routine and should ideally last for at least ten minutes. Stage 5 is an excellent way of dealing with the fears and anxieties of antenatal depression, so you should study this stage before you begin. Alternatively you can make a tape of yourself reading the words and relax to this.

Stage One
• Lie in a comfortable position and repeat the breathing exercise from the start of this routine.

Stage Two
• Once you feel centred, visualise a warm flow of air rushing up your spine with each inhalation.

Stage Three
• As you exhale feel any tension or stress disappearing down your spine and out of your body.

Stage Four
• Focus on each area of your body starting with the feet, ankles, calves, thighs and buttocks, then moving on up to your hands, arms, shoulders, neck and head. This breathes in warmth to these areas and breathes out any tension or stress.

Stage Five
• Now concentrate on the area around your navel. As you continue to breathe deeply think about your baby being soothed by your breathing. Picture the baby nestled inside you and feel proud of what you have achieved. Let all negative thoughts and emotions leave your mind and focus on the wonder of creating the new life inside you. If fears and worries do pop into your head acknowledge them and let them drift away again. Then send a message of love and warmth to your baby. You have nothing to fear – what is happening to you now is the most natural process in the world. Think of your baby growing stronger day by day, preparing for the process of birth. Feel your baby draw-

ing strength from you and feel strengthened in return. Forget all about any fears for the future – enjoy your present state of total relaxation – just you and your baby, bonding and growing together.

- Take as long as you like on stage 5. When you are ready to get up, gently rotate the wrists and ankles to wake the body up slowly.
- Rub the palms of your hands together and place them over your closed eyes. Open your eyes and slowly slide your hands down your face. Then roll on to your side and gently push yourself up into a seated position.
- Stretch your arms up overhead, gently reaching for the ceiling and inhale deeply. Exhale and return your arms to your sides.

Exercise and Postnatal Depression

If you are suffering from postnatal depression the chances are that the very last thing you feel like doing is any form of exercise. You are probably exhausted and feel you have scarcely enough time to look after your baby, let alone look after yourself. However, taking care of yourself is often the key to breaking free from depression and regular exercise helps in the following three ways:

- **By regulating the brain's mood neurotransmitters.** Studies have shown that 30 minutes of aerobic exercise (any activity that leaves you breathless) will improve the mood and lower anxiety levels for several hours afterwards. Carried out on a regular, long-term basis, this form of exercise can make a lasting impact on depression.
- **By accelerating weight loss.** A common cause of distress following the birth of a child is that the excess weight put on during pregnancy does not disappear overnight. The stomach that was once pulled tight around your unborn baby now flops down in a huge blubbery fold. And as for your breasts – their gravity-

defying days seem well and truly over! It is not surprising that many women feel a sense of despair when they find themselves still wearing maternity clothes and afraid to look in the mirror several weeks after giving birth. The good news is that by following a regular exercise programme it will take much less time to lose this excess weight than it did to put it on. Once your body begins to take it's old shape and tone you should also start to regain your self confidence.

• **By increasing energy levels.** Believe it or not, exercise actually increases energy levels and raises stamina. By exercising you will find it easier to cope with the new demands placed upon you and your feelings of helplessness should, hopefully, start to diminish.

Before you start

Your body undergoes a huge transformation during the nine months of pregnancy and this should never be underestimated. Hormonal changes cause the ligaments to soften, posture is altered by excessive weight gain and giving birth itself can lead to various physical complications such as tender scar tissue from an episiotomy or caesarean section. All these factors need to be taken into consideration before embarking upon any type of exercise programme. The length of time since the birth and your previous level of fitness also have to be taken into account, but one thing is certain, if you are suffering from postnatal depression it is never too late to start exercising.

What kind of exercise?

For the first six weeks after the birth you should avoid any kind of strenuous aerobic activity as your body needs time to recuperate. However, a gentle programme of stretching and relaxation, targeting the specific muscle groups that have suffered most, such as the stomach, waist, legs, back and the pelvic floor, will help speed up the recovery process, both mentally and physically. Try the yoga programme in the previous section, remembering not to force any of the positions – if you feel faint or have any pain stop immediately. Once six weeks have passed, and as long as you are not suffering from any physical complications, you can widen your range of exercises to incorporate some form of aerobic activity. Again, listen to your body and only do as much as you feel able. Another important thing to remember is to choose a type of exercise to suit the way you are feeling. If you are particularly tired there is little point in forcing yourself to go for a three-mile run when a relaxing yoga routine would be so much more beneficial.

Some of the common excuses for not exercising

'What's the point? I can hardly be bothered to get dressed most days, let alone keep fit.'

Initially keep it simple. Walk rather than taking the car or bus and then feel proud of this achievement. Aim to walk for at least 20 minutes every other day and then increase this target to every day. When you feel able, slowly start to introduce other forms of exercise, such as a gentle stretching session twice a week. Focus on what you are actually doing rather than what you could be doing.

'I only had two hours sleep last night. How am I supposed to have the energy to exercise?'

A simple yoga routine, with its gentle stretching and deep breathing techniques, is easy to do when tired and will actually leave you feeling refreshed and invigorated. Even a short walk around the block will lift your spirits when you are feeling drained.

'How can I take regular exercise when I am tied to my baby 24 hours a day?'

- Purchase exercise videos or books or devise your own programme to do at home at your own convenience.
- Going for a jog is invigorating and also gives you a welcome sense of freedom if you are feeling chained to the house. It is also

easy to fit into your schedule as you are not restricted to a set time or day and you only need to leave your baby with somebody else for a short period of time.

• Buy a customised stroller and take your baby with you for a brisk walk or jog around the park. This should reduce levels of irritability and stress in both of you.

• Once your baby has completed her first set of immunisations you will be able to take her swimming. If you make this a family event you will be able to do a few lengths while your partner minds the baby. Once again, by including your baby in your exercise routine you will benefit not only from your own improved mood but also from a relaxed and sleepy baby.

Relaxation Techniques for Antenatal and Postnatal Depression

Sufferers of both antenatal and postnatal depression experience high levels of stress, anxiety and even panic attacks. By practising a combination of relaxation, visualisation and breathing techniques you will learn to control these symptoms of your depression and minimise their impact. When we are under stress our bodies hunch up and our muscles clench tight. Practise frowning and see how hard the muscles in your face have to work. Now relax your face into a smile. It requires so much less energy for our bodies to relax and yet when we are depressed total relaxation is the hardest thing in the world to achieve. Practise the following relaxation exercises and techniques and put them to use at times of stress and anxiety.

Basic tense and relax technique

This is a very simple way to achieve a complete state of relaxation, for mind as well as body. It can be cut short to focus on specific areas of tension when you are short of time. For example, you may like to focus on just the arms, shoulders and face immediately after feeding your baby to remove instantly any tension that may have been caused.

- Lie down in a comfortable position in a quiet place away from distractions (if circumstances do not allow this, the technique can also be practised in a comfortable seated position).
- Take four deep breaths in and out through your nose and be aware of your diaphragm rising and falling.
- Curl the toes up as tightly as you can, hold for a second and then let them relax.
- Now push your feet away from you as hard as you can without moving the rest of your body. Hold and push and then allow your feet to flop outwards, completely relaxed.
- Next clench your calf, thigh and buttocks muscles, push them down into the ground or chair beneath you, hold and then allow your legs to fall open to a comfortable, relaxed position.
- Now move up to your abdomen. Pull your stomach muscles in tightly, pressing your back down into the floor, hold and then relax.
- Clench your fists into a ball, press your arms in tightly to the sides of your body then allow your arms and fingers to fall open and relax down once more.
- Raise your shoulders up to your ears in an exaggerated shrugging motion. Hold for a few seconds and then allow your shoulders to fall back down.
- Finally, clench your face up into a frown, tighten your jaw and wrinkle your forehead. Hold and then slowly allow your face to relax completely. Let your mouth fall slightly open, relaxing your jaw, let your eyelids become heavy and imagine any remaining tension draining out through a hole in the top of your head.
- Now focus on your breathing which should have become increasingly shallow. Only inhale as much air as you require and then exhale fully. Remain in this relaxed state for as long as you require. You may like to listen to some soothing music or alternatively you may like to practise a visualisation technique.

Visualisation

This exercise is an excellent counter for feelings of stress or negativity. Once you have practised it a couple of times it will become
increasingly easy to slip off into your own secret, visualised world
when you need to escape from the pressures of reality. This exercise should leave you feeling far more relaxed and positive about
yourself and your situation.

- Relax in a comfortable position away from any distractions.
  You may like to follow the basic tense and relax procedure of the
  previous exercise. Alternatively, lie down and allow your arms
  and legs to fall apart as far as is comfortable from the body, with
  palms and toes upturned.
- Be aware of how open you feel as you focus on your breathing,
  in and out, slowly and steadily through your nose.
- Allow all the barriers you have built up around yourself to melt
  away, and concentrate on feelings of love and warmth.
- Now visualise yourself walking through a field. Be aware of the
  rhythm of your feet upon the ground, slow and steady.
- Picture yourself arriving at a door. Open the door and step inside.
  You have arrived at your own special place; it could be deep in
  the heart of a forest or floating down a stream. Enjoy building up
  the picture of this place in your own imagination. Let your mind
  run free. What do you hear in this place? What can you smell?
  How do you feel? Make this place completely your own – it is
  your retreat from all of your problems and worries. Here you can
  only feel warmth and contentment. Here you are carefree and
  confident. Picture yourself laughing and full of vitality.
- When you are ready to leave, visualise yourself slowly walking
  back through the door and into the 'here and now'. Become
  aware of your surroundings and the position of your body.
- Slowly rotate your wrists and ankles.
- Take a couple of deep breaths and rub your hands together.
- Place your palms over your eyelids and slowly open your eyes.
  Slide your hands down your face and back to your sides.

- Take a big stretch, inhale deeply, and then gently ease yourself back into a seated position.

Simple stress-relieving exercises

Any form of stretching exercise will help you to relax, but at times of stress it is not always physically possible to launch into a full-blown yoga routine. Here are some quick and easy tension-relieving exercises that can be slotted into your daily routine as an instant antidote to stress.

Shoulder stretches

Exercise one

- Sitting in an upright position or kneeling on the floor, interlace your fingers and place them at the back of your head with your elbows facing out to the side *(see illustration 17)*.

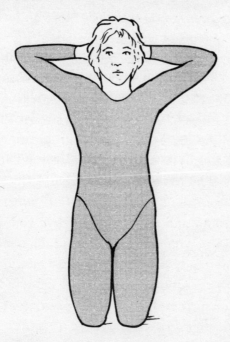

Illustration 17. *Shoulder stretches. Exercise 1. Interlace your fingers and place them at the back of your head with your elbows facing out to the side.*

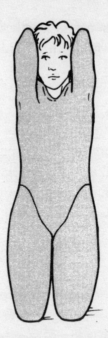

Illustration 18. *Shoulder stretches. Exercise 1. Pull your elbows in towards your face.*

- Staring straight ahead of you inhale deeply through your nose and pull your elbows in towards your face *(see illustration 18).*
- Exhale and return your elbows out to the side.
- Turn your face to look upwards and repeat the exercise, remembering to breathe correctly.
- Finally repeat the exercise with your face looking down and your chin tucked in towards your chest.

Exercise two

- Seated in an upright position inhale deeply and shrug your shoulders right up to your ears.
- Hold the position and hold your breath for a few seconds.
- Exhale deeply and relax the shoulders back down.
- Repeat several times.

Exercise three

- Place your hands on your shoulders and take it in turns to circle each shoulder backwards and then forwards.

- Then repeat with both shoulders together.
- Complete this exercise with both shoulders down in a relaxed position.

Breathing

When we are under pressure our breathing immediately becomes quick and shallow. By taking deeper, slower breaths you will instantly diffuse any tension building up in your body. Practise the following exercises as a way of controlling your breathing and encouraging relaxation.

Exercise one

- Sit in a comfortable position with your spine extended and head up, eyes gently closed.
- Breathe in through the nose for a count of two.
- Hold the breath for a count of two.
- Exhale through the nose for a count of two.
- Repeat this exercise increasing the length of the count by one each time.
- When you reach the highest count with which you are comfortable (this number will increase with practice) start to work your way back down, reducing the count by one each time, until you get back to a count of two.

Exercise two

- Sitting in a comfortable, upright position breathe in through your nose for a count of four and then exhale for four. Repeat a further three times.
- Fold the middle three fingers of your right hand into the palm, keeping your thumb and little finger outstretched.
- Bring your left hand up to your nose and block the left nostril with the left thumb (see illustration 19).
- Inhale and exhale for a count of four, four times through the left nostril.

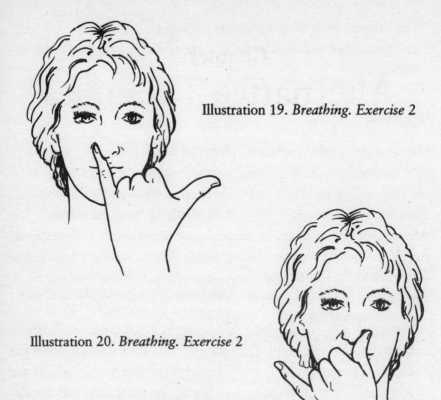

Illustration 19. *Breathing. Exercise 2*

Illustration 20. *Breathing. Exercise 2*

- Then swap sides, blocking the right nostril with the little finger of the left hand, breathing through the right nostril four times *(see illustration 20)*.
- Breathe in through the right nostril, then block that nostril with the thumb and hold the breath for a count of four.
- Slowly release the little finger and exhale through the left nostril.
- Inhale through the left nostril, then bring the finger up to block it once more and hold your breath for a count of four.
- Release the thumb from the right nostril and exhale.
- Continue breathing in through one nostril and out through the other four times.
- Then return to the start of the exercise and breathe in and out through both nostrils four times.

Chapter 9
Alternative Therapies

Alternative therapies are an increasingly popular form of treatment for depression. However, before using complementary treatments for antenatal or postnatal depression there are two key points to bear in mind.

- **Harmful side-effects.** Very little research has been carried out regarding the effects of different alternative treatments upon the foetus. There is a common misconception that herbs and oils are a natural, safe alternative to chemically manufactured antidepressants, but this is not always the case. Many of the herbs and oils used by alternative practitioners are extremely powerful drugs and during pregnancy should be treated with the same caution as conventional medication. It is *vital*, therefore, that sufferers of antenatal depression consult their doctor or a qualified practitioner in complimentary medicine before undergoing any form of alternative treatment.
- **The severity of the depression.** Sufferers of postnatal depression do not face the same potential health risks from alternative therapies. However, for sufferers of severe depression it is important to view complementary medicine as exactly that: 'complementary', and to use it alongside more conventional forms of therapy or antidepressants for the most effective results.

As long as you bear these points in mind there is no reason why the wide range of alternative therapies on offer cannot play a key role in your recovery.

Herbal Treatments

St John's Wort

St John's Wort, a herbal treatment for depression derived from the Hypericum perforatum plant, is often referred to as 'nature's Prozac'. Available over the counter in most health food shops and chemists, it is widely accepted as an effective treatment for moderate cases of depression. In 1996 the British Medical Journal published a report summarising the findings of over 20 different studies carried out on St John's Wort, concluding that it was just as effective as most other antidepressants, but with fewer side-effects. The active ingredients, called hypericins, affect the mood-altering chemicals within the brain in a similar way to Prozac, but in a less invasive way. Occasionally it can lead to minor side-effects, such as stomach upsets, and heightened sensitivity to the sun in fair-skinned people. The usual recommended dosage is 900mg a day and it should begin to take effect within 2–3 weeks.

Sheryl began taking St John's Wort when she was still suffering from postnatal depression ten months after the birth of her daughter Kylie:

> *'I was becoming desperate to get back to normal, but I just wasn't able to shake off this sense of doom and gloom. On the face of it I had absolutely nothing to feel depressed about – I had three healthy children, a loving husband and a nice home, but for some unexplained reason I felt really down. It was like I was going through the motions of my life, unable to experience any kind of emotion, just this sort of numbness. I read about St John's Wort in a magazine and I decided to give it a go. I liked the fact that I could buy it over the counter and not have the embarrassment of going to my doctor. I didn't notice any change at first, which was a bit of a disappointment – I think I had been hoping for a miracle cure. However, after about three weeks there was a slight improvement. Slowly I felt my energy returning, I had more patience with the kids*

and I was less irritable with my husband. I wouldn't say that St John's Wort alone cured my depression, but it certainly got me back on the right track. Life didn't seem so hopeless any more and it became easier to feel more positive.'

For further information contact the Hypericum Information Centre (see Useful Addresses section at the end of this book).

St John's Wort and antenatal depression

Unfortunately, as there has been no detailed research into the effects of St John's Wort upon the foetus, most experts in complimentary medicine are very reluctant to recommend it to pregnant women. Although it has fewer side-effects than other antidepressants, St John's Wort is still a powerful drug and will be transmitted from the expectant mother to her unborn child. You must seek advice from your GP before taking any form of medication whilst pregnant.

Aromatherapy

Aromatherapy uses pure plant extracts in oil form to treat various different ailments including depression and other related problems such as exhaustion, insomnia and anxiety. Widely available in health food stores, chemists and various other shops, the oils come in two forms: essential and aromatherapy. Essential oils are very potent and need to be diluted with a base oil (such as almond). They should be stored in a cool, dark place, out of the reach of children and never put neat on the skin. Aromatherapy oils are bought ready-diluted with a base oil. The aroma from these oils can be released through massage, when diluted in the bath or when vaporised in oil burners or room sprays.

Aromatherapy and antenatal depression

As with herbal treatments there is a real danger in assuming that the oils from plants cannot possibly harm the foetus. This is, however, far from the case. Some oils are in fact extremely dangerous during pregnancy, in particular **basil, clary sage** and **rose. Lavender oil** should also be avoided until very late in the preg-nancy or until the birth itself. The following oils are considered safe for use during pregnancy and can be very effective in treating the various causes and symptoms of antenatal depression:

Panic attacks, palpitations and rapid breathing – ylang ylang, lemon balm
Nausea – grapefruit
Fatigue – grapefruit, lemon, lime, orange blossom, peppermint
Depression – peppermint, and towards the end of the pregnancy, lavender

However, as with all forms of treatment during pregnancy it is best to seek professional advice before using aromatherapy oils. For further information contact the International Society of Professional Aromatherapists (see Useful Addresses at the end of this book).

Aromatherapy and postnatal depression

After you have given birth there is a far wider range of oils available to treat depression and its associated symptoms:

Anxiety – basil, geranium, ylang ylang, lemon balm
Depression – clary sage, lavender, melissa, rose with insannia, vetiver, peppermint
Insomnia – lavender, mandarin, melissa, vetiver
Relaxation – bergamot, frankincense, lavender, rosewood

Acupuncture

Acupuncture is an ancient form of Chinese medicine and one of its integral parts. It works on the basis that the body has an invisible network of pathways known as meridians. A type of energy known as qi (pronounced *chee*) flows through these pathways. When this energy becomes blocked or unbalanced the belief is that it will result in some form of illness, either physical or mental. Acupuncture is designed to unblock the pathways and restore and rebalance the flow of qi. This is achieved by painlessly inserting tiny needles into the skin at various points in the body. In the treatment of depression the needles are used to work on the nerves sending messages to the brain. This in turn is believed to make the brain release endorphins (our body's natural painkillers and muscle relaxants) increasing our sense of well-being. Acupuncture is also thought to have an effect upon the limbic centre in the brain (the part responsible for mood and behaviour). It is the most widely accepted form of alternative therapy and is even practised by some GPs.

Acupuncture and antenatal depression

Acupuncture is quite safe and can be used as early as six weeks into the pregnancy. However, as with all forms of treatment it is advisable to consult your doctor first and to ensure that your practitioner is properly qualified. There are two main organisations for qualified acupuncturists. The British Acupuncture Council (BAaC) is for practitioners who are not medically trained. They will have MBAcC after their name. The British Medical Acupuncture Society (BMAS) has members who are fully trained doctors.

Acupuncture is an excellent form of treatment for the sufferer of antenatal depression as it can help with all of the following different problems encountered throughout the pregnancy.

First trimester (after six weeks)

Morning sickness – acumagnets (magnetic patches) can be purchased to place over the acupuncture points to quell feelings of nausea.

Early pregnancy bleeding

Migraines

Fatigue

Second trimester

Heartburn and indigestion
Fatigue
Haemorrhoids

Third trimester

Backache and other aches and pains as your weight increases
Carpal tunnel syndrome
Sciatica
Labour pains

By using acupuncture to treat chronic nausea, and as a potential form of pain relief during the birth, sufferers of antenatal depression can alleviate two major sources of stress and anxiety. As acupuncture can also be used to treat depression, insomnia and general anxiety it forms a perfect all-round treatment and is well worth looking into.

Acupuncture and postnatal depression

In cases of postnatal depression, acupuncture will target all of the symptoms associated with depression: stress, anxiety, insomnia, as well as any potential hormonal imbalances. For further information contact the British Acupuncture Council (see Useful Addresses section).

Flower Remedies

For centuries, flowers have played a large part in healing all around the world, but it wasn't until the 1920s that a British Harley Street physician named Dr Edward Bach reintroduced them to the West. Dr Bach (pronounced *Batch*) had begun to identify mental stresses and anxieties as being at the root of many physical ailments and he wanted to find a suitable treatment for these psychological causes of illness. It was really due to intuition that he first began experimenting on flowers and plants, but over the course of the 1920s and 1930s he developed a total of 38 different flower remedies.

Flower remedies are made by leaving freshly-picked flowers to float in spring water in warm conditions, allowing the essence of the flower to be transmitted to the water. This water is then mixed with brandy as a preservative and stored in a dark glass bottle. A few drops of this essence is then slowly sipped in a small amount of still mineral water. Flower remedies are believed to lift the mood and overcome negative feelings at an energy level rather than chemically, making them totally safe and free from side-effects. However, there is no accepted research into their effectiveness and they are probably best used in conjunction with other forms of treatment such as counselling, rather than in isolation.

Different flowers are used to treat different symptoms, but they can be mixed if you are suffering from more than one of the following:

Depression – gentian, gorse, sweet chestnut, wild oat, wild rose
Anxiety – agrimony, aspen, cherry plum, mimulus, red chestnut, rock rose, vervain
Fatigue – hornbeam, olive

Most health food stores stock a wide range of flower remedies and there are many books available on the subject. For further information contact the Flower Remedy Programme (see Useful Addresses section).

Massage

Massage is a well-known stress reliever and undoubtedly benefits the sufferer of antenatal depression by easing away feelings of stress and anxiety (albeit on a temporary basis). More recently, massage has also been shown to help women suffering from post-natal depression. A small study carried out at Queen Charlotte's

Hospital in London found that sufferers of postnatal depression who attended an infant massage class began to develop closer relationships with their babies. As difficulty in bonding seems to go hand-in-hand with postnatal depression, infant massage appears to be an effective way of minimising the impact upon the child as well as helping the mother. For further information on infant massage see your GP or midwife.

Conclusion

Just as there are many potential causes of antenatal and postnatal depression there are many different treatments on offer. However, the first step in any successful recovery will have to come from within yourself. No matter how many books you read or how much love and support you receive it is ultimately down to you to acknowledge that you have a problem and to be brave enough to seek help. This is by far the hardest part in conquering depression. You must not feel guilty or punish yourself if all you feel like doing today is sitting on your own and crying . The time will come when something inside you says, 'enough is enough', and you will take the first tentative step down the road to recovery. Whether this involves seeking help from your GP or midwife, phoning a helpline or even buying this book – once you have made that first crucial step things should slowly start to fall back into place.

When I wrote my first article on antenatal depression I had no idea just how widespread the problem was. What began as a curiosity as to what went wrong with my own pregnancy, resulted in me discovering that I was far from being alone. I had never imagined that what I went through actually happens to 10 per cent of all pregnant women. I had also never imagined that the stress I was under could potentially harm my unborn child and lead on to postnatal depression. Having a child should be one of the most joyful experiences of a woman's life, but as many as 20 per cent of women are finding it one of the most frightening, anxious and stressful of times. The health service is beginning to address the problem of postnatal depression with increased publicity and more emphasis being placed on a new mother's mental as well as physical health, but in at least one-third of cases this is just shutting the stable door after the horse has bolted. How much unnecessary pain and suffering could be avoided if women were offered adequate support and information from the beginning of their pregnancy rather than being left alone to suffer in silence and shame?

During the course of researching and writing this book I have spoken to and received letters from countless women who had been through or were still suffering from antenatal or postnatal depression. These women came from all kinds of backgrounds and situations, but the one thing they had in common was their traumatic experience of pregnancy and birth. From the chronic anxieties to the deep despair and overwhelming sense that they were alone, their stories were extraordinarily similar. However, once on the road to recovery, many of these women found that they had been left with an overwhelmingly strong bond with their baby. It was as if, having finally found their way out of the darkness, they were literally dazzled by the love they discovered for their child, as the following diary extract reveals:

'I have never known such happiness, such completeness. I never want it to end. They tell me, "Don't pick him up when he cries", but they don't understand. How can they? How can they know that there was a time when he was ignored, unwanted, his arrival dreaded, his future uncertain? For all I know he probably sensed all the hostility I felt towards him, so God knows how insecure he must have felt. Now he's finally here and all's well, nothing is too much for him; not feeding, attention, cuddles or love. Just being with him is such peace, such total peace.'

Useful Addresses

Alcoholics Anonymous
Tel: 0845 769 7555

Association for Postnatal Illness (APNI)
25 Jerdan Place, London, SW6 1BE
Tel: 020 7386 0868

British Acupuncture Council
63 Jeddo Road, London, W12 9HQ
Tel: 020 8735 0400

British Association for Counselling
1 Regent Place, Rugby, CV21 2PJ
Tel: 01788 550899

British Association of Psychotherapists
37 Mapesbury Road, London, NW2 4HJ
Tel: 020 8452 9823

British Medical Acupuncture Society
60 Great Ormond Street, London, WC1N 3HR
Tel: 020 7278 1615

British Wheel of Yoga
Central Office, 1 Hamilton Place, Boston Road, Sleaford, Lincs,
NG34 7ES
Tel: 01529 306 851

Flower Remedy Programme
PO Box 65, Hereford, HR2 0UW
Tel: 01873 890218

Gingerbread (for single parents)
49 Wellington Street, London, WC2E 7BN
Tel: 020 7240 0953

The Hypericum Information Centre
PO Box 5810, Brackley, NN13 7ZD
Tel: 01280 709877

The International Society of Professional Aromatherapists
ISPA House, 82 Ashby Road, Hinckley, Leics, LE10 1SN
Tel: 01455 637987

La Leche League International (for information on breast-feeding)
Box 3424, London, WC1N 3XX
Tel: 020 7242 1278

Meet-a-Mum Association (MAMA)
58 Malden Avenue, South Norwood, London, SE25 4HS
Tel: 020 8656 7318

Mind (National Association for Mental Health)
22 Harley Street, London, W1N 2ED
Tel: 020 8519 2122

National Caesarean Support Network
c/o Sheila Tunstall, 2 Hurst Park Drive, Huyton, Liverpool,
L36 1TF
Tel: 0151 480 1184

National Childbirth Trust
Alexandra House, Oldham Terrace, Acton, London, W3 6NH
Tel: 020 8922 8637

National Council for One Parent Families
255 Kentish Town Road, London, NW5 2LX
Tel: 020 7267 1361

Refuge (for women in abusive relationships)
See phone book for the number of your local branch

Stillbirths and Neonatal Deaths Society
28 Portland Place, London, W1N 4DE
Tel: 020 7436 5881

Twins and Multiple Birth Association
PO Box 30, Little Sutton, South Wirral, L66 1TH
Tel: 0151 348 0020

References

Chapter 1

1 Walther, V.N. (1997) 'Postpartum Depression: A Review for Perinatal Social Workers', *Social Work Health Care*, 24(3–4): 99–111

Chapter 3

1 Nott, P. et al (1976) 'Hormonal Changes and Mood in the Purperium.' British Journal of Psychiatry 128: 379–383
2 Harris, B., Lovett, L., Smith, J., Read, G., Walker, R. and Newcombe, R. (1996) Cardiff puerperal mood and hormone study. III. Postnatal Depression at 5–6 weeks postpartum, and its hormonal correlates across the peripartum period. British Journal of Psychiatry. 168: 739–744
3 Whitton, A., Warner, R. and Appleby, L. (1996) 'The Pathway to Care in Postnatal Depression: Women's Attitudes to Postnatal Depression and its Treatment.' British Journal of General Practice 46 (408): 427–428

Chapter 5

1 'Glover, V., Teixeira, J., Gitau, R., Fisk, N.M. (1999) 'Mechanisms by which Maternal Mood in Pregnancy May Affect the Foetus', Contemporary Reviews in Obstetrics and Gynaecology, published by the Foetal and Neonatal Stress Research Centre, Imperial College School of Medicine, Queen Charlotte's and Chelsea Hospital
2 Pawlby, S. et al. Taken from an article in the Observer newspaper entitled 'Postnatal blues can lower IQ of baby boys' (23/1/00) in which it details the most recent research carried out in this area and says 'the researchers are to publish their work in the Journal of Child Psychology and Psychiatry'. At the point of publication there was no volume no. available.

Chapter 6

1 Walther, V.N. (1997) 'Postpartum Depression: A Review for Perinatal Social Workers'. *Social Work Health Care*, 24 (3–4): 99–111

Index

irrationality 44
isolation 4, 70–1
IVF 52–3

Jane's story 2–3
Japan, attitude to childbirth 70
Jennifer's story 37–9
jogging 153–4

labour, fear of 18–19
lemon chicken and hummus 121
lethargy 4, 41
limbs, tingling in 42
loneliness 69
lunch and light meals 120–4

madness, feelings of 21
magnesium 109–10
main meals 124–7
massage viii, 167–8
meatloaf 125
medical help 84–100
Melanie's story 63–4
memory loss 44
mental health, fears about 21
milk of magnesia tablets 109
mineral and vitamin supplements 110
miscarriage 14–15, 64
Moira's story 58–9
mood, improvement with exercise 151
mood swings 11
morning sickness 6–7, 106–11
mother, pressures on 16–17, 39–40
mother, relationship with 56–7
moving house 65
muesli 117
multiple births, fears about coping 20–1

National Childbirth Trust 71
nausea 6–7 see also morning sickness
nervousness 41
Nicola's story 3
nightmares 42
nutritional deficiencies 101–2, 103–6, 112

oestrogen 5, 46
Olivia's story 39
over-sensitivity 41

panic attacks 42
paranoia 44
parenthood 16–17, 30
parents, conflict with 4
partner
  abusive 61
  anxiety about 17–18
  and depression vii–viii
  effects of depression on 72–8
  unsupportive 60–1
Paul's story 59–60
phobias 42
physical causes of depression 4–11, 46–55
Pitt, Professor Brice 36
plans, for the future 97–8
porridge 117
possessiveness 4
postnatal depression 36–71 see also antenatal depression; depression
  and diet 112–15
  effects on baby 81–83
  causes 46–71
  how to avoid 28–34
  link with antenatal depression 27–35
  symptoms 42
postnatal exercises 34, 152–4
postpartum psychosis vii, 37, 44–5, 100
pregnancy
  fears about baby's health 19–20
  first-time 12–13
  and nutritional deficiencies 103–6
  physical complications 10–11
  unplanned 14
  and work 22–3
premenstrual syndrome and depression 46–7
professional help, fear of 85–6
progesterone 5, 46